WEIGHTLESSNESS

Integrated Exercise: Yoga, Pilates, and Chi Kung

WEIGHTLESSNESS

Integrated Exercise: Yoga, Pilates, and Chi Kung

RAY RIZZO

iUniverse, Inc.
Bloomington

Weightlessness
Integrated Exercise: Yoga, Pilates, and Chi Kung

Artistic Director/layout and graphic design by Boramy Thong (www.bothong.com)
Photos: David Arraez (www.davidarraez.com)

All images are the author's calligraphy and are based on ancient Taoist healing symbols, signifying longevity and liberation, except for illustrations listed in the resource section. These images are licensed as Public Domain and used in accordance with the GNU Free Documentation Act.
See appendix for a full list of illustrations.

iUniverse books may be ordered through booksellers or by contacting:

iUniverse
1663 Liberty Drive
Bloomington, IN 47403
www.iuniverse.com
1-800-Authors (1-800-288-4677)

Because of the dynamic nature of the Internet, any web addresses or links contained in this book may have changed since publication and may no longer be valid. The views expressed in this work are solely those of the author and do not necessarily reflect the views of the publisher, and the publisher hereby disclaims any responsibility for them.

ISBN: 978-1-4620-4163-3 (sc)
ISBN: 978-1-4620-4164-0 (e)

Printed in the United States of America

iUniverse rev. date: 12/29/2011

IN•TE•GRAT•ED adj.*

1. Made up of elements or parts that work well together.

2. Bringing together processes or functions that are normally separate.

3. Open to everyone, without restrictions based on race, ethnicity, religion, gender, age, or social class.

Microsoft Encarta Dictionary.

" I hope martial artists are

more interested in the root of martial arts

and not the different decorative branches,

flowers or leaves.

It is futile to argue as to which single leaf,

which design of branches,

or which single flower you like;

when you understand the root,

you understand all its blossoming."

—Bruce Lee

CONTENTS

ACKNOWLEDGMENTS

I would like to extend my appreciation to my friends and clients, as their patronage allowed me to develop these ideas; to my family, Ron, Holly and Carina; to my teachers, Dharma Mittra, Lazaro Ayesteran, Simone Felice, Ehren Hanson, David Pakenham, Steve G.; to Coy Smith, Sharon and Jeff Feinstein, Frank Doblecar, Dan Stone, and the Gregans; to David Arraez for his photography; to Defne Duna for the last minute Pilates advice; to Nick Fitzwilliams; to Boramy Thong for his generosity and artistic genius; and to Dara Thong, whose love rescued me from the "jungle."

PREFACE

When I tell someone that I teach yoga, very often their next question will be, "What style of yoga do you teach?"

Ah, well, it's complicated. I practice the healing arts—yoga, chi kung, Pilates, acupressure, and manual therapy—but I have never been overly concerned with one particular style or teacher. Instead, I have sought internal experience through practice. I have studied with masters in China, India, and New York; with Sufis in Istanbul, shamans in Peru, and osteopaths in France. My motto is—as Bruce Lee once said, paraphrasing Sun Tzu—"study everything you can, absorb what is useful, and discard the rest."

With that as a guiding principle, this book began to take form, first as notes, then as sequences of exercises derived from the evolution of my own practice, formal education, classes, and private sessions. I remember the manuscript's first incarnation as a spiral-bound workbook; a friend leaned over and said, "It will take about ten years to finish." He was right.

Indeed, the journey from conception to American publication has been a long one. This book was first published in Europe, and then translated to Turkish and Russian. Since then, I have had the opportunity to deepen my practice, allowing these forms to continue to evolve while teaching them around the world and integrating the feedback from my readers. The book itself has gone through several incarnations, and I am grateful to all those who have helped along the way.

I suppose it's a style; but without techniques, without forms, what do you teach?

Note: The pronoun "he" has been used instead of "he/she." This is not meant to exclude the female gender and is employed solely for linguistic efficiency. I also use the older spelling of chi kung, which is now spelled qigong in pinyin, the current system used to translate Chinese characters into roman letters.

—Ray Rizzo

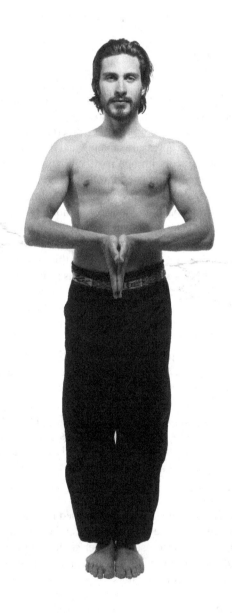

INTRODUCTION

We live in a world that bears witness to an explosion of ideas, scents, foods, clothes, cars, travel, books, and media. The challenge is no longer to acquire information—as it was in the days before globalization—but rather to sift through the chaos and find what really works. The same is true when it comes to mind/body systems such as yoga, Pilates, and chi kung. Some are quasi-religious, others purely physical. Every one seems to have a name, a brand.

Many people have asked me about different styles, about the comparative benefits. *Which one do you think is the best? What style do you teach?* My answers are often elusive: All styles are really one. The most important thing is practice. Authentic learning.

Nevertheless, in the midst of all the body and mind disciplines and styles, there are a few forms that are more inclusive and not so differentiated or specialized; they focus on the essence of movement. They challenge strength, flexibility, awareness, balance, and many other faculties simultaneously. *Weightlessness* is a synthesis of these forms. The movements, stretches, postures, and meditations in this book can be grouped together under the title *Integrated Exercise*. Their common goal is the optimization of the human instrument.

Ultimately, this program is designed to enhance, rather than compete with or replace the singular styles such as the Pilates method, old-school chi kung, or any of the various schools of yoga. The purpose is to connect you to the language of your physique and to provide an easy-to-learn set of exercises that can be done on a daily basis, in your own home, and with little discipline. The exercises are accessible to people of all fitness levels, simultaneously simple enough for beginners and challenging enough for advanced practitioners.

If the body is an instrument, this book is a study of its scales and chords. Mastering these—your chops, so to speak—enables you to play any song. These forms are safe and multi-applicable, challenging, yet also meant to support a restorative, healing practice. Most of all, they are selected to give us the strength and grace to walk through this life. Keep in mind, these are not just exercises for physical fitness. The real goal is the application of intelligence—learning how to learn.

For me, yoga is the fine calibration of the human instrument for optimal expression of intelligence and creativity. It is a path to freedom. If you want to do it professionally, then you may want to learn advanced postures like splits and inversions, to study the literature and scriptures, and adopt a vegetarian diet. But for many people, it is not relevant to learn Sanskrit mantras or practice complicated breathing exercises. It's not about becoming a yogi *per se* but about improving our health and awareness.

So here we are, with our bodies, our scars, our wounds, and the parts we love and hate. Here we are with the vessel that we have counted on to digest our food, carry us to the market, and to rally us through pleasure and pain. Here we are, resident in a being of infinite subtlety and complexity—some of the most incredible neurological, chemical, biological, and consciousness-based systems on the earth—and yet this organism has now been bombarded with 20, 40, 70, 90 years on this crazy planet. Sprained ankles, chicken pox, car accidents, lost loves; the body carries a kinesthetic index to it all. Yoga is the liberation from this memory.

Have you ever had a great night's sleep, and woken up bright-eyed, alert, and feeling light? What about another day, maybe it is raining outside, your neck is stiff, and you can barely get out of bed? That's life, we say, but the fact is we all need a way to help keep the stress of reality from weighing us down. In other words, by the time we turn off and tune in, most of us are already pretty banged up. What happened? And more importantly, what can we do about it?

I always assumed that we were born in balance and it was the world that caused us to go out of tune. Then, after more than ten years of teaching yoga and healing arts, my first son was born. He was a healthy child and well formed but had a severe contraction to one side, going down from his neck to stomach and hip. A mild contraction (torticollis) is common, and most people think it goes away, but what I learned as I began observing babies, is that it doesn't really disappear. Since birth, many of us are born with subtle asymmetries that stick around for life and often will come back with a vengeance in old age. Almost all my clients who are over thirty have some visible distortion; by sixty, the patterns are setting in. But many of these problems could have been prevented if each joint had been systematically opened, understood, and restored.

You want to get in shape? There are a few ways you can go about it. You can build strength on top of fundamental imbalance—muscles get bigger, and you can lift more weight. Or you can build power on harmony—your muscles become more efficient, and you improve your quality of life.

The fact is that we are designed symmetrically, but life is asymmetrical. The goal is to restore symmetry to our lives. Getting involved in personal transformation means you go directly to the source and increase strength and range of motion simultaneously. Again, let's consider the human body as an instrument: playing sports is like playing a song, *integrated exercise* is tuning the instrument, practicing the scales and the chords. A finely tuned instrument can make anything sound good.

The transformation is difficult, but the results are worth the investment of time and labor. If you're disciplined, focused, and committed, you will become renovated, renewed, and rejuvenated.

You wake up one day and say, "Today I will change my life," which can take six weeks or six months or sixty years. It's a gradual process. During this period, you must be humble, watch your diet, and stay the course. But it's not enough just to hit the mat or the gym. You must relearn how to walk, dance, and drive. You go joint by joint. How does my wrist move? How do I stand on my feet? Why do I lean so much on one leg? You examine your old movement pathways and make new ones. You've got to be vigilant, watch out for corruption, and carefully observe your sensory feedback. I recognize it feels like a daunting task, but when you consider the alternative—your body rotting slowly—isn't it worth it?

TRANSFORMATION

Are you free? I wasn't. When I was eight years old, I would swing on vines with my friends. We were like little monkeys. One day, we found a vine that swung out over a cliff, very high, and it was a big rush for our boy pride. I slipped off the vine that day. I remember reaching for branches as I fell 5, 10, 20 feet down. I cracked open my head, suffered a good concussion, and received a lot of stitches. It took months to heal, and when I thought I was completely better, I noticed a lingering pain and stiffness in my neck, shoulders, and lower back. That pain persisted for almost ten years.

What did it feel like? I felt trapped. If someone held me down and stretched me, it would cause fear—fear of the unknown, fear of the tension and irritability, fear of my anatomy. By the time I went to college, I had become accustomed to the headaches and other nagging remnants of the injury. But it wasn't just the injury acting upon me; it was a combination of factors. My body was calling out for me to map it and build an infrastructure; it was coffee, sugar, anger, cigarettes, postures, attitudes, bad nights, break ups.... All these end up heaped on top of our skeletons. My mind and body, though relatively young and healthy, were so far from where they needed to be.

It's a matter of cause and effect. The tension that had built up in my muscles and joints was there because I had never opened my body; I had never learned to tune my instrument. I had learned to do my taxes, to brush my teeth, to change the oil in my car, to do the dishes, to balance the checkbook, to play sports, to pay attention. But no one had ever shown me how to heal my body or to align and maintain the most precious thing I owned. Walking around in a stupor,

slouching at the table, having bad knees and shoulders up by my ears, a stiff neck... there came a moment when I said, "That's it; I want everything out!"

I began to study yoga and started a lifelong quest for optimization. I was hooked; hooked on taming the wild, irritable impulses, on creating symmetry and beauty, but most importantly, ease. Somehow, it seemed that as my body opened, so did my heart and mind. I was about to realize that I was the owner of an internal realm, an undeveloped paradise that was storing more energy than I could have imagined.

On a daily basis, I would stretch with the essential postures of yoga. My first breakthroughs came with the forward bend. I could almost *hear* my formerly untapped energy stirring as I felt the taut wires of my neck gradually releasing. I remember also, after months of doing yoga, the first time I could comfortably grab my feet. It was almost like déjà vu; the last time I could do that, I must've been a child. Suddenly, nothing could be more important than striving for optimization, the harmonious development of all human faculties—physical, spiritual, emotional, intellectual. Thus begins the transformative phase.

Within three months of beginning my practice, I had completely rid myself of the headaches and the neck and shoulder tension that had plagued me for ten years. I realized that yoga was more than just exercise, and I started reading everything I could about it. I felt I had come out the other side of a tunnel. *Welcome to the bright world.*

It was around this time in my progression that I became familiar with what is known as sacred geometry as well as the advanced mathematics of fractals. To sum it up, there are some essential mathematical formulas for shapes, distances, and growth patterns that repeat themselves all throughout the world, like a universal blueprint. A cat's paw, DNA, a ram's horn, hurricanes, fingerprints, and the spiraling Milky Way galaxy—all might be reducible to a fundamental equa-

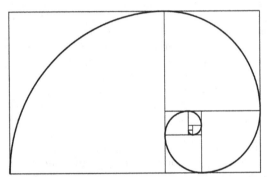

The Golden Spiral

tion, the *golden mean* or ratio, aka the Fibonacci sequence. What if there was such a thing at the root of all human movement? There had to be. This book is the result of the quest for that oracle.

In my search for the most efficient and effective practices, I soon became interested in the study of gymnastics. The gymnast who I first trained with was from Cuba. At thirty-six, he was remarkably chiseled and able to flip his body with ease. I wanted to learn the back flip, and in courting that muse, he took me through the fundamentals of movement. Before each session, we would complete a warm-up. It was

on these summer nights that I began to notice he was teaching me the basic elements of connecting with my body. Not as poetic as chi kung, as specific as yoga, nor as linear as Pilates, here was the simple essence. Here was the road map and infrastructure that I would need to excel in any sport and to integrate any martial art. Also, here was a familiar language that could be safely communicated to just about anyone. I took careful notes, and a year later, after completing my training in Pilates and therapeutic massage, I opened my first studio.

Something woke up inside of me. I wanted to find a way to study learning itself, so that I could open many doors with one key. While completing my bachelor's degree in consciousness studies at the State University of New York, I practiced handstands, flips, rock climbing, trapeze, and swimming. I trained in balance, responsiveness, agility, flexibility, speed, awareness, and timing—while extending key insights to my friends and clients. Through it all, I noticed there were some very consistent themes at the base of all these traditions and I began to get a sense of *Weightlessness*—the relaxed state of ease that accompanies the liberated body and mind.

Then, while taking a sabbatical from my studio, I entered the Peruvian Amazon to participate in a traditional shamanic apprenticeship, called a *dieta.** It was there, deep in the jungle, that I finally developed the four sets of exercises that would become the core of this book. Those were some of the happiest days of my life—except for one thing; I couldn't wait to get out into the world and begin my work.

---

* For a more detailed description of this experience, please see the Afterword, "Shamanic Yoga." A dieta involves several weeks of fasting or a diet of simple foods such as plantain and rice. It also utilizes silence, herbal baths, and the ingestion of medicinal plants such as Ayahuasca.

HOW TO USE THIS BOOK

Weightlessness is about exercising, yes, but most of all it is about connecting with a feeling: embodied transcendence. We can't always change the reality of the planet—suffering, struggle, hunger. But we can do something to keep it from entering our bodies and weighing us down. It is a personal quest, not about saving the world, but about liberating ourselves. We must, above all else, remain uplifted.

The book is divided into four parts. Part one begins with a chapter called "The Weightless Zone," which outlines the meaning behind the movements. Next comes "The Breath." People often ask me when to breathe in, when to breathe out. In the beginning, it doesn't always matter. What matters is that you breathe. After this comes "The Basic Warm-Up," designed to loosen the sinews and lubricate the joints.

The next three parts correspond to three sets of exercises. These form the backbone of the integrated exercise language. Part II, "The Maintenance Set: Exercises for Ease" is accompanied by a DVD (available at www.rayrizz.com or on Amazon) to demonstrate the basic forms. It includes my versions of the "Eight Brocades," a classic chi kung exercise, the "Sun Salutes" from yoga, and the "Swimming Dragon" (also from chi kung). These exercises should be accessible to everyone, including children, the elderly, and women in the early stages of pregnancy. Each part of this set takes only about ten minutes; think of it not so much as working out, but as preparing you for life. These are the main exercises that I developed and practiced in the jungle of Peru.

Part III, "The Therapeutic Set: Postures of Rest and Rejuvenation," covers ways of restoring the body–mind relationship. It teaches you how to turn the body off and find serenity. It also includes troubleshooting for common ailments, such as a stiff neck, sciatica, and carpal tunnel syndrome. Certain components of this set can be practiced daily, as part of a bedtime ritual, for example.

And Part IV, "The Advancement Set: Exercises for Mastery," covers hatha yoga, Pilates style exercises, and various elements from mixed martial arts. These exercises may not be appropriate for everyone, so you must gauge your abilities and remember to practice safely. The exercises can be used as a full Pilates or yoga workout, or separately to target specific areas. They can also be used as a reference or to enhance your participation in other classes. If you are in good shape, try to do the exercises from this set two or three times per week.

The final chapter, "Self-Observation," goes a bit deeper into what it means to train awareness and human faculties, and explores the different states of consciousness. This is followed by an Afterword on "Shamanic Yoga." Though I have studied traditional methods, I choose not to practice yoga only in its ancient forms. I teach what I know, and my approach to spirituality is as much influenced by the time I've spent in the jungle, as it is by Sufi poets like Hafiz and Rumi, and by the work of Joseph Campbell. I don't speak Sanskrit; instead, I live in a global age and have chosen to incorporate other symbols from diverse traditions to show the common themes with regard to the quest for optimal attunement of the human instrument.

In the beginning, focus on the exercises in the maintenance set. I recommend you try to do at least one form every day. Whichever makes you feel the best. Then try one set in the morning and one in the evening. Take your time, because ten minutes of focus is more helpful than an hour of mindless thrashing. Ideally, for your daily maintenance, you would do the warm-up or the Eight Brocades, as well as a few Sun Salutes, and four Swimming Dragons. That's my personal recipe. But, by all means, play, discover, invent, and feel.

Shoot for every day; then, even if you only practice three to five times per week, it will still change your life. And please don't be daunted by the number of exercises in this book. Learn the maintenance set, make it a part of your life, and expand from there. At the end of some of the following chapters, there are key ideas and concepts to ease your understanding. The reader may notice that some sayings are simple and others more abstract; use them as meditations and insights to accompany your practice. Try to allow the suggestions to work on multiple levels: rational, intuitive, and physical.

Weightlessness is your guide, but you are the trainer, the guru, and the master. It is up to your mind, your focus, and your inspiration; it is up to you to take your energy and invest it in yourself. You are it, and I personally guarantee that the rewards are greater than any external boon, real estate, or stock. When you begin to feel yourself appreciate, your whole reality changes.

INTEGRATION

There is an old saying that goes like this: Before enlightenment, a man looks at a mountain and says, "It's just a mountain"; during the process, he says, "It is trees and ecosystems, climate, and watershed"; after enlightenment, he says, once again, "It is just a mountain." The same is true for your body—it is designed to function perfectly, but in order to create that state of ease you have to undergo the transformative phase, a journey back to vitality. During this phase, you will need the help of teachers and the exercises in this book. Once you have fully restored your health, all that will be necessary is a minimum daily practice.

I wish you well on the journey of reintegration. We are equipped with the start-up package. Now it's time for the upgrade. Integrated Exercise is based on this premise: all major muscles in the human body are technically voluntary, but in reality, we have little control over many of our parts. Your practice is the process of creating a fully conscious and optimized being. The only way out is through.

As you reintegrate, you may notice you have some objective limitations—hard facts that aren't going to change. But you must realize also that there is almost always a huge margin for real improvement. You may notice that parts of your body have been asleep, numb, shut down, and neglected. Use frostbite as an analogy: you don't feel it when you are out in the cold, but when you come inside, it stings. That burn is the pain that lives in the body as it is released. It is the power of your circulation returning. Likewise, as you begin to unlock your body you may become aware of aches and pains that had long since been locked away. Stick with it, and the pain disappears.

Sometimes people ask me if it gets easier, and I say yes, easier to express joy. Muscles that do not compete against each other are exponentially more effective; the joints have more stability and last longer. And if form follows function, then it is also true that the most useful muscles are the most beautiful. They are the ones that express the chiseled vitality that we all adore.

All forms are derived from the essence. It is my hope that you will use this program to help you connect to your own inspiration, to your own genius and intelligence. Most of what you really learn comes not only from certifications or workshops or schools, but from constant practice, self-observation, and awareness—from hard battles won in the mythic wilderness of your own mind. The ancient yogis and sages all learned from watching nature. The many forms of kung fu and chi kung are named after the sets of movements that animals make—tiger, monkey, praying mantis, horse, crane, and so on. And just as the human fetus passes through all the stages of evolution before becoming *Homo spiritus*, all the wisdom of the universe is in your cells, in the spine, in the limbs, and in the mind. What's more, when you learn from your own inspiration, no one can take it from you. It is authentic, hardcore realization.

You can change your body. In the beginning, you have to fix up the instrument. You have to adjust the strings and straighten the neck. Once all is in place, all you have to do is tune and play. Likewise, as your body gets more aligned, the maintenance will be minimized and then you can get to the good stuff, which is life. The irony is that it is actually easier to build an efficient body than to build one that is simply strong. It takes less time, fewer repetitions on fewer machines, but it takes more focus. You've got to show up. Awareness is the key.

You are about to embark on your own quest. There may be little wilderness left in the world; many of the natural predators may be dead or tamed, and temples may have become like museums, but the internal battle—the wilderness between your ears and inside your skin—is just as perilous and mythical as ever.

The goal is to slay the ogre and recover your spine, to trick gravity and earn the great boon, *WEIGHTLESSNESS*.

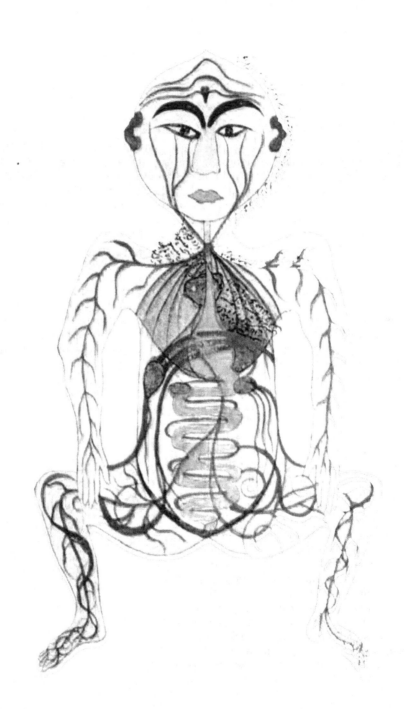

PART I

STARTING IN:
DEVELOPING YOUR FOUNDATION

Chapter 1. *The Weightless Zone*

After you read the following paragraph, please take a moment to stand up. Now feel the weight on your two feet. Do you lean more to one side? What about your hips and pelvis? Is your back relaxed? Your shoulders? Your neck? What if you close your eyes and rock forward and back slightly. Imagine that gravity is a hand pushing down on your head. What happens?

If you are aligned, that hand will push directly through you and down to the earth, but when you are out of alignment, it begins to throw the body out of whack. Maybe it pushes the head forward like a hunchback? Or makes the neck bend? Now try to find the point where you are just in balance, where you feel perfectly centered, as if you're not falling forward or back. Imagine you are a scale; seek the zero point.

This is the *weightless zone*. And it has little to do with gaining or losing a few pounds. It is about the experience of being. About opening the spiritual heart. When you move from this center—which I will also refer to as the *circle of ease*—all movements will be graceful. Why? Because you are removing the friction and drag from the body. Essentially, you are learning to float. To be in the moment with presence and awareness. This is what it means to be in center.

This chapter will outline some of the universal myths and symbols that relate to the concept of centering. But first, let's take a moment to review the human form.

ANATOMY OF BEING

After birth, we are equipped with locomotion, digestion, elimination, and basic kinesthetic awareness. That's the start-up package. The other software has to be downloaded. When it comes to learning the language of the body, the basics can be learned in a few sessions, but you can spend a lifetime mastering the subtleties.

The purpose of this chapter is not to teach the specifics of anatomy and physiology. It is more important that you understand on a deeper level simply how to move with ease. The world offers a wealth of information on muscles, bones, Latin names, and exact functions. What we are focused on is how to free the body and awaken internal energy. Understanding this comes naturally when you begin to observe your way of interacting with space. The trick is to engage with your body's intelligence and process what it tells you—listen to your joints. In other words, *explore, understand*, and *feel*.

Many of us have problems with slouching, atrophy, and asymmetry. We have muscle groups that overwork and those that underwork. Coming to alignment—or centering—means that you start really paying attention. From this awareness, you can begin to intelligently distribute your energy. How do you know when you're off-center? Perhaps there will be pain or discomfort; joints may click and pop. When this happens, stop! Return to the weightless zone and start to move again, slowly and carefully, until you find the *circle of ease*.

It helps to find a guru or teacher—guidance speeds things up in any learning process—but the most important thing is that you learn to listen to your body, to become sensitive and able to discriminate between the real and the false intuitions. Whether you have a teacher or not, the most important voice to listen to is within. As you reconnect with your body, you must be aware of all habitual movement. For example, how are you sitting right now? The challenge is to develop new patterns and bring mindfulness to each action. Beginning with the spine ...

CHI AND THE CENTRAL NERVOUS SYSTEM

At the center of it all is the vertebral column, housing the brain and central nervous system. The spine consists of roughly thirty-three vertebrae and is broken down into five regions: the cervical (neck), thoracic (mid-back), and lumbar (lower back) regions, plus the sacrum (pelvic region) and coccyx (base of the spine or tailbone). Additionally, there is the cranium or skull.

The hard skull and thick bones of the vertebrae are all designed to protect the brain and spinal cord, which acts as the go-between from the senses to the cerebral cortex. The keystone of the skull, near the top of the spinal column, is a hang-glider shaped bone called the sphenoid, and the pituitary gland sits right in the center of it, like a pilot. The pituitary gland is responsible for the regulation of the rest of the hormonal (endocrine) system. Behind the pituitary sits the pineal gland, which many see as the seat of visualization. To the ancient yogis and seers, optimal health was not the end goal, but just the means to enhanced spiritual awareness and, ultimately, to the attainment of a state of union (with self or God or all of creation). By activating this visionary mechanism of the human brain, the obstacles to full realization of the energy of the universe could be removed. Physical optimization is one way of activating this gland.

Many cultures have believed there is a force that animates us and electrifies the brain and central nervous system; they have sought techniques such as breathing, exercise, and meditation to awaken this force and have it rise up our spines, to purify and strengthen the body so that it can express our inner intelligence and create a feeling of expansion. In many traditions, we see this represented as the second birth, the awakening of internal energy, the cultivation of a conscious human from the automaton (from *Homo sapiens* to *Homo spiritus*), and so on. Beyond health, this is the common goal of yoga, Pilates, and chi kung.

Central to all three disciplines is the concept of *chi*, or in the Indian tradition, *prana*. These are two different names for what is essentially the same concept, usually translated as *life force energy*. If you are adverse to "spiritual terms," then you can think of it as bioelectricity, or the body's electromagnetic field. Basically, we are alive, and then we're dead. Something left? That something is chi.

Though chi is currently difficult to prove or measure, science has been able to identify the electrical transmissions across synapses in our nerves. The rest of the body, including the bones, muscles, respiratory, digestive and circulatory systems are basically just the casing for the central nervous system or neurovegetative* entity, which communicates along pathways or meridians.

While the Indian tradition often considers chi or prana to be coiled in the base of the spine, the ancient Taoists believed it was concentrated in the core. In martial arts, this is known as the *dan tien*, *hara*, or *inner sea*. All things radiate from the center out. The strength of the strongest limb is nothing compared to the core. When energy comes from the core, it integrates multiple body and

---

Autonomic nervous system.

mind zones. This is the difference between strength and power.

Anatomically, a strong core is made up of a "woven" abdomen. We'll call this the snake belt. It is a combination of the *iliopsoas* muscles, the *quadratus lumborum*, and the abdominals. The superficial muscles (the six-pack) work together with the muscles on the side and the back to form a postural base—like the four walls of a foundation. This group of muscles is designed to harness the energy of the spine, the central intelligence. And also to hold us up. From there, it branches out to the hips, the shoulders, the arms, the legs, the feet, and the hands. Sound familiar?

Our bodies are organized in symmetry. The limbs are the same on either side, so really, if you understand one, you understand the other, and this provides valuable information. The shoulder girdle (rotator cuff) distributes the energy from the core to the arms. The hip cuff distributes the energy from the core to the legs. The neck flexes forward and laterally, rotates and extends. As you begin to practice, attempt to make the two sides even, generate chi from the core and the spine, position the limbs with the shoulders and hips, and deliver intention through the hands and feet.

The postures and movements are like an electric tuner that gives us information about the state of the human. That's why it is so important to seek maximal efficiency. Archimedes said, "If you give me a lever and a place to stand, I can move the world." Likewise, when we use the right muscles at the right times, our bodies become much more efficient, with far less effort and strain, freeing us up to move the world within.

Traditional yoga and chi kung take the position that anatomy and physiology are informed by our state of mind and our awareness. The process of integration is the process of consciously creating the body, regulating the mind, and finding a state of ease. At the top of the pyramid all sides come together; at the pinnacle of awareness, the body is kept in perfect form.

THE CHAKRA SYSTEM

The ancient rishis (yogic seers) conceptualized the human energy field in terms of two currents and the human being as the magnetic conductor between the cosmos and the earth. When we are fully aligned, we are a conduit, not a shelf. The subjective experience of gravity shifts, leaving us with a feeling of buoyancy; the skin, bones, and organs stay healthy and energized.

Energetically, the spine can be thought of as two interwoven serpents, or a double helix. One current of energy rises up, the other descends. In classical Indian philosophy, this energy is known as *kundalini*, or the serpent of the spine. This energy is the currency, the electricity, and the force of moving intelligence.

The S-curve of our spines can also be understood as a conduit for the magnetic and electrical energies of the universe. When these two are balanced, there is harmony. If one of the waves is out of balance, it creates dissonance; this is where weight and tension accumulate.

According to this philosophy, the ascending and descending currents enter the body through the nostrils and intersect seven times (some say eight, including one that is outside the body). Each locus, or point, is called a *chakra* (wheel).

The first chakra (Muladhara) is at the root of the body, between the groin and the anus. This is vital to survival. It relates to our simple essentials—food and shelter. The second chakra (Swadhisthana) is just below the navel and represents sexuality, specifically procreation. The third chakra (Manipura) is located below the diaphragm and is tied to will, activity, and competition.

Man has the first three chakras in common with the rest of the animal world—survival, sex, and hierarchy. The fourth chakra (Anahata), which relates to compassion, is where it becomes interesting. Animals feel fear, love, and other emotions, but arguably none has this truly human quality of compassion, which means "to suffer with." If you transpose a cross over the chakra diagram, it intersects at the fourth chakra—what is known in many traditions as the spiritual heart.

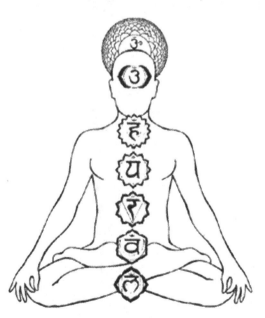

Mythically, the virgin birth in Christian tradition can be thought of as the awakening of what is truly human out of the animal. This is because our animal-self gives birth to the higher self or divine being; the act of lifting the spine against the hand of time is an immaculate conception, a metaphor for resurrection. In this brutal world, the act of self-actualization and transcendence is a lightning bolt of beauty that can add personal meaning to an otherwise hostile existence. It all hinges at the fourth chakra. From there, the two currents can unite heaven and earth.

The fifth chakra (Vishuddha) relates to communication and belongs to the realm of art and poetry; it is found in the throat area. The sixth chakra (Ajna) relates to the third eye, and represents vision, reason, and inspiration. The seventh (Sahasrara), at the crown of the head, opens to the cosmos and connects us to the infinite wisdom of the universe.

Each chakra relates to emotions, colors, organs, glands, and planets. The more we stand upright and unlock the power of the spine, the more we float through life, and the less the hand of gravity pushes us down. When aligned correctly, the two currents of energy can connect with each other, plugging us in to the energy of the universe. Ultimately, the chakras are not just "spiritual centers," but tools in helping us to understand the different motivations in the human being. The upper chakras are dependent on the lower ones to function. While some of the ancients insisted on an extremely austere lifestyle—minimizing the pull of the lower chakras—the point of view of *Weightlessness* is not to exclude the lower chakras in order to become only *spiritual*, but rather to align and tune the entire being in order to become *fully human*.

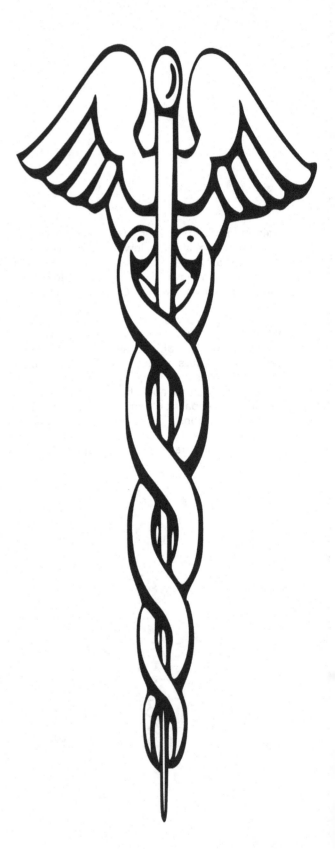

ALCHEMY AND ASTROLOGY

In our own Western tradition, the ancient seers spent endless hours observing the stars. Astrology was once an essential part of interpreting the significance of events. Man had his place within the universe. He wasn't separate from it, and it wasn't something he could control. The trick was to find a way of submitting to and aligning with the energy of the universe. Music, poetry, and the healing arts sought to reflect and emulate this mystery. As above, so below. The ancients believed that if you were silent and conscious enough you could hear the sounds that were emitted from the seven visible orbs (planets), and these sounds—the music of the spheres—became the basis for the seven octaves. There are seven cervical vertebrae in the neck, roughly the same in the sacrum (which means sacred). When the musculoskeletal system is properly tuned—capable of holding the subtle rhythms of tension and relaxation that bring about a quality of grace—it literally resonates with the music of the spheres, bringing about radiant health, improved mental clarity and even psychic abilities. When this occurs, a human can know his purpose, if nothing else, as an instrument in the terrific and fascinating orchestra of the cosmos.

THE WINGED SPINE

Many cultures have used a tree-of-life motif to represent our innate intelligence. It can be found in certain Kabalistic (Hebrew mysticism) diagrams as well as in Egypt, Greece, Africa, and the Near East. The caduceus and Asclepius's staff have even been adopted as the symbols of Western medicine, as a kind of fusion between the tree of

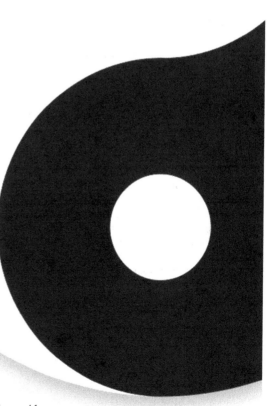

life and the double helix. The caduceus,* or staff of Hermes, is depicted as two snakes wrapping themselves around a staff. Four sevenths of the way up—at the crux of the cross and the compassion center—these snakes sprout wings. It is a paradox, a flying serpent. The bridge between heaven and earth. Why would the East and the West both choose the serpents as the symbol of medicine?

Throughout mythology, the serpent is a symbol of immortality. The serpent possesses the ability to shed skins, which to primitive man was the same as being reborn. These symbols far predate our understanding of the genetic code and the structure of DNA, but perhaps this discovery was anticipated. Both DNA and the two interwoven serpents share the same structural identity. Is this merely a coincidence? Or does it relate to the structure and power of the human central intelligence system?

These symbols were originally associated with Hermes, and later with medieval alchemists. But the alchemists weren't just looking to turn lead into gold. In reality, they were attempting to turn the base, innate behaviors in man—the lusting, craving animal—into the spiritually ascended being. Indeed, if you consider what separates us from all the other animals on the planet, it is the fact that we stand upright—hence the name of one of our hominid ancestors, Homo erectus—and therefore we have the capacity to unite the ascending and descending currents. The plumed, or winged, serpent is a universal symbol of the alchemized being. When you connect to the energy of your spine, and learn to push the hand of gravity, it is as if the snake (spinal column) sprouts wings, allowing the base elements of the human being to soar to transcendent heights. And it simultaneously charges the organism with subtle energy.

---

*The caduceus is Hermes's staff (two serpents) and is meant as a magic wand for commerce, often mistakenly used for medicine; Asclepius, the god of healing, had a staff with just one serpent, and it is the one used by the AMA, and the correct medical symbol.

MERIDIANS

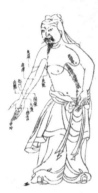

In Chinese medicine, the energetic currents branch throughout the body in twelve major lines of energy called meridians, plus two auxiliary channels. Each line connects to emotions, glands, energies, and organs and corresponds to one of the five elements: earth, wood, water, metal, and fire. Acupuncture and acupressure work with these pathways and the relationships of the elements to restore the body to a state of ease. Chinese medicine recognizes that in addition to the chemical, neurological, and biological components that are essential to life, the human being is also an electrical and magnetic presence. Health is a matter of the uninterrupted flow of these bioelectrical forces, or chi.

The yin-and-yang symbol is essential to our understanding of meridians and Chinese medicine. Again, it displays two currents—one ascending, one descending—united as pairs of opposites. Beyond that duality is the great ultimate or Tao. Where Western exercise often focuses on the building of muscles, strength and appearance, the Taoist system seeks an optimally attuned being, with a balance between the active and the passive, the strong and the flexible. As the old saying goes, "be rigid like the oak tree and you will snap in the heavy wind, be flexible like bamboo and you can bend and sway".

BODYMIND

A bit of universal mythology can help put in perspective the miracle of the vessel that carries us around, and it gives a metaphysical overview for us to orient our practice. From the chakras to the Hermetic staff to the Star of David to the Christian cross intersecting at the heart, many of the world's "religious" symbols have had a sense of the sacred geometry of the human form. Across the board, the snake—therefore the spine—recurs as a symbol of immortal life.

Until recently, despite its awe-inspiring discoveries, the field of medicine still deemed it heretical to suggest that consciousness could play any role in healing the human body. And so all studies were based—despite results showing significant placebo effects—on proving a double negative: It doesn't not work. It was strictly off limits to engage the patient's intelligence. But if sugar pills (placebos) can cure diseases a significant portion of the time,* then there must be something in the power of the mind to influence the material or physical form. Studies to test the efficacy of medicines and treat diseases have tremendous value, but a philosophy that concentrates on disease alone is not sufficient for the practice of health.

Movement therapies, along with advanced bodywork (osteopathy/acupressure) can help create the conditions for health by working on four important levels. The first is the muscular level, which can be treated by massage. Second is the neurological, which can be treated by acupressure/acupuncture. Third is the level of bone, treated by manual adjustments, similar to chiropractic. Finally, in addition to prescribing medicines to treat symptoms, it is important to engage the intelligence of the human being, the conscious entity. This is the shamanic or psychotherapeutic level. When all four levels are engaged, it becomes possible for real healing to occur on all levels, because you are jumpstarting the body's innate intelligence.

A recent study identified the power of chi kung to aid in the recovery from a certain type of cancer.* All participants were given the same anti-cancer drugs, but only one group participated in chi kung exercises and guided visualizations. Ultimately, the exercise group far exceeded the control group in terms of recovery and sense of well-being, with a 32 percent improvement over the patients that received drug therapy alone. This shows how the body is not distinct from the mind as previously thought; rather, the mind can potentially contribute to healing of even hard-to-treat diseases.

This integrated approach is sometimes referred to as body-mind medicine, meaning that the human being is seen as a whole that is greater than the sum of its parts. Body-mind medicine attaches importance to hard science as well as to feelings and thoughts. It accepts that a human being is a two-way street: sensations are running from the senses to the brain and also from the brain or mind to the senses. When the body is aligned, at peace, and integrated, the immune system can function optimally, exhibiting a type of force field that is really just optimal health. Most of us have probably heard the saying "the body is a temple." And all these disciplines, both in their physical as well as metaphysical forms, are seeking to unite us with the divine energy of the universal consciousness.

Many yoga poses and chi kung mediations focus the energy on the pituitary gland, or third eye. The intention is to stimulate the immune system in order to maintain healthy endocrine (hormonal) function. Sickness is caused by pathogens, but because we are constantly bombarded with disease-causing agents, we get sick because of a chink in the armor, a hole in our defense system. A real cure eliminates the symptom and then goes to the source of the weakness. It is one thing to treat the effect—the tumor, the broken knee, the cough—another thing to treat the whole person. Both are necessary.

When you discover the circle of ease, you must go there as often as possible and stay there as long as possible. These exercises are not just about building muscle definition or weight loss. They are alchemical formulae designed to lift the body, to inspire. By practicing yoga, you can bring your senses under control. When the mind becomes a clear mirror, then you can see yourself. That's what we came here for. All the great wisdom traditions have maintained that we are more than just cells, tissues, and neurochemicals. When we lift our spines and remove the physical obstacles from our lives, we begin to enjoy weightlessness, attunement to the rhythm of the cosmos. Keep these notions in mind as you begin your practice. In this way, exercise can be approached not just as preventative medicine, but also as a sort of nondenominational prayer. A way of showing up and reckoning.

---

* Michael Haederle, *The Placebo Effect: Studies Reveal How Fake Medicine Actually Reduces Pain,* http://www.alternet.org/health/144327.
* Kevin Chen, PhD, MPH, and Raphael Yeung, BA, *Exploratory Studies of Qigong Therapy for Cancer in China,* http://www.flowingzen.com/science.html

SOLAR PLEXUS MEDITATION

The solar plexus is located near what is called the "spiritual heart," in the center of your torso, just to the right of your physical heart. It is the point of light where the lower, third chakra has given "birth" to the higher, human elements of the fourth chakra. The mystical states of alignment, nirvana, and nondualistic union are founded and grounded in the liberated body; their sacred overtones are in the vertebrae, the mystical hormones of the master glands, and the intelligence of the cerebral spinal fluid. The sacrum, the sphenoid, the gut, and the crown, all are laid out like resonant octaves, at one with the music of the spheres.

Sit in meditation position or rest on your back and feel all seven chakras line up. Focus on the cross that intersects at the heart chakra and notice the top of your head pushing up. Visualize the spine as a double helix of light, a magnetic and holographic energy field. Lengthen the space between each of your vertebrae, particularly those in the neck. Breathe gently through each one. Feel your diaphragm begin to fill, not just with oxygen, but also with the cosmic prana. Life force. You might feel a light just below your sternum, but if you don't, don't worry, you will once you have mastered subtle breath techniques. This is the solar plexus, where you will awaken your true breath-power.

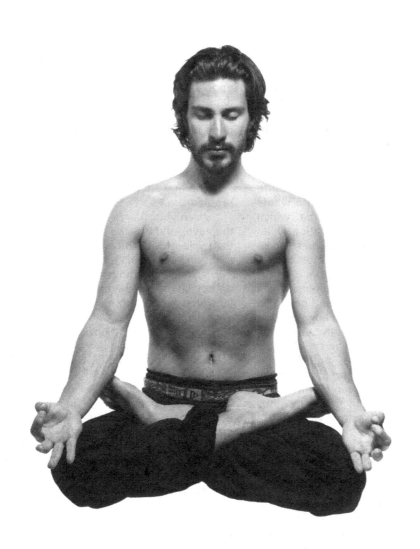

Chapter 2. *The Breath*

Y ou can engage in many different exercises: you can jog, do gymnastics, practice yoga, Pilates, and lift weights ... but what is most important is to cultivate your awareness. It is not a question only of strength, weight-loss, or cardio endurance, but a question of grace, weightlessness, and serenity. The first and most important key to mind and body well-being is the breath. Breathing is the primary means to control the mind, nourish the chi, and synchronize internal organ rhythms. There is even a whole branch of yoga known as *pranayama*, which deals with the mobilization and activation of life energy, *prana*. But again, it's not always necessary to do a lot of exercises. What is most important is that you simply learn to breathe.

Let's begin at the beginning. Imagine for a moment the birth process. We are floating in watery bliss, fed, oxygenated, and enveloped in the only world we know. Suddenly, there is a tremor, followed by waves and shivers, the doctor's sterile hand guiding us out, and finally, a smack on the back and our first breath, followed by tears. As we cry, we fill our lungs with air for the very first time—a simple yet miraculous process. But as life progresses and we begin to acquire character armor as a result of traumas and injuries and in the forms of emotional postures and stress compensation, the body often becomes rigid and locked.

All this is connected to the breath.

Whether we are overweight or rail skinny, strong or atrophied, whether we exercise five times a week or five times a decade, chances are we have fallen into any number of degenerative breathing patterns known as reverse breathing. What is reverse breathing? Simply put, it is a shallow breath that allows the abdomen to drop like a fallen soufflé. Reverse breathing is the opposite of the anatomical function singers, dancers, and martial artists tell us is right. It is responsible for any number of postural distortions leading to rigid spines, distended organs, weight gain, back pain, and sciatica; it leads to muscular tension, lack of vitality, and an overall life posture of *I give up*.

The first step to recovery is to recognize the problem.

Place your hands on your belly, right above the navel, and breathe naturally. First, just notice the cycle of inhalation and exhalation. At what point do your hands move out?

If your belly moves in and your chest rises on inhalation and the belly drops on the exhalation, you are breathing without properly using your diaphragm.

You are breathing upside down.

REENGAGING THE ABDOMINALS WITH DIAPHRAGMATIC BREATH

Change is a process, but until we learn to breathe, all other exercises are relatively useless. If you can feel the right sensation, even just once, there is hope. Fortunately, there is a very simple way to work toward breaking this breathing pattern: "When in doubt, cough it out."

Place your hands on your abdomen—now cough. Do you feel the muscles contract? This cough is an exaggerated version of what is called a *forced exhalation*. Because it is an uncorrupted, unconscious reflex, it circumvents the mind and allows us to reconnect to the first deep breaths we took in the delivery room. It is the beginning of relearning the most efficient and healthful way to breathe.

Relearning how to breathe is simple and, with practice, will once again become an involuntary act. It is, after all, the natural, life-enhancing way to breathe, and your vitality will rapidly show you its merits. *All you have to do is fill up and empty out from the diaphragm.*

The diaphragm is a flat, somewhat concave muscle that attaches just under your ribcage. It is shaped like a shallow cone. It divides the lung and heart region from the rest of the organs, such as the liver, kidneys, and intestines. When it functions properly, it massages these vital organs and also helps them to remain correctly positioned.

On a more spiritual note, the diaphragm divides the body's lower three chakras (energy centers) from the upper, which is to say it is a metaphysical paradox, separating yet uniting what is animal from/to what is spiritual in each of us. It is so central to our existence that certain breathing techniques are the foundation of the "rebirthing" therapies that guide people through the visceral memories associated with birth trauma. In order to know yourself, breathing is the place to start.

We are now going to learn the essential steps to diaphragmatic breathing, also known as D-Breath.

Ancient Yogic Parable

Once upon a time, the five senses and the breath got into an argument about who was the most important. Finally the brain said, "Each of you go away for one day, and we'll settle this."

First, the eyes went away, and the body bumped into a few things and had trouble walking, but that was all. The ears left, and everyone missed the sounds of the birds.

When the sense of touch left, the body felt lonely. Smell went away, and there was little inspiration for the stomach and a strange loss of memories. Finally, taste went away, and food had no flavor.

When all of the five senses had returned, the breath went away. After just a few seconds, the eyes cried, the nose ran, the skin tingled, the tongue curled, and the ears began to pound. The brain couldn't think at all and yelled out, "Come back, come back! Do you think this is a joke? You are killing us."

The breath returned, and everyone knew who was the king.

1. The Basic Stance

We'll begin in the Basic Stance.
Stand with your feet shoulder-width
apart and distribute your weight
evenly over ball, toe, and heel. Take
a moment to make sure your legs
are in line. Then bend your knees
slightly and align the shoulders,
hips, and ears.

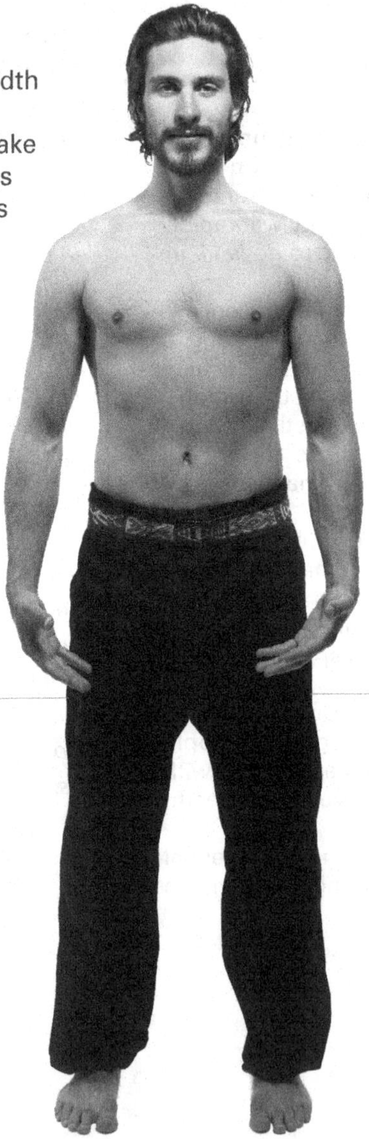

Fig. 1: The Basic Stance

⦿ Imagine that gravity is a hand
  pushing down on your head.

⦿ Try to align everything so that the
  energy passes directly through to
  the earth.

⦿ From the waist up, let the vertebrae expand.

⦿ From the waist down, allow all
  energy to drop to the earth.

2. Diaphragmatic Inhalation

Place your hands on your belly. Take a medium-size breath in while keeping your chest steady but allowing your abdomen to expand. When you have fully inhaled, your belly should be out.

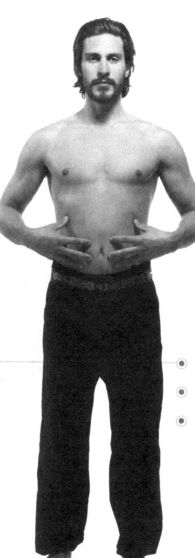

Fig. 2: Diaphragmatic Inhalation

- Allow the belly to fill with air.

- Keep the chest steady.

- Only inhale three quarters of the way.

3. Diaphragmatic Exhalation

Lay your hand lightly over your diaphragm. Cough. Cough again. Can you feel the forced exhalation? This is what you want to practice but in a more subtle and controlled fashion. Use the abdominals to squeeze your breath out, but do not allow the energy to push you back; instead let it lift you. Imagine your breath expanding the space between each of your vertebrae.

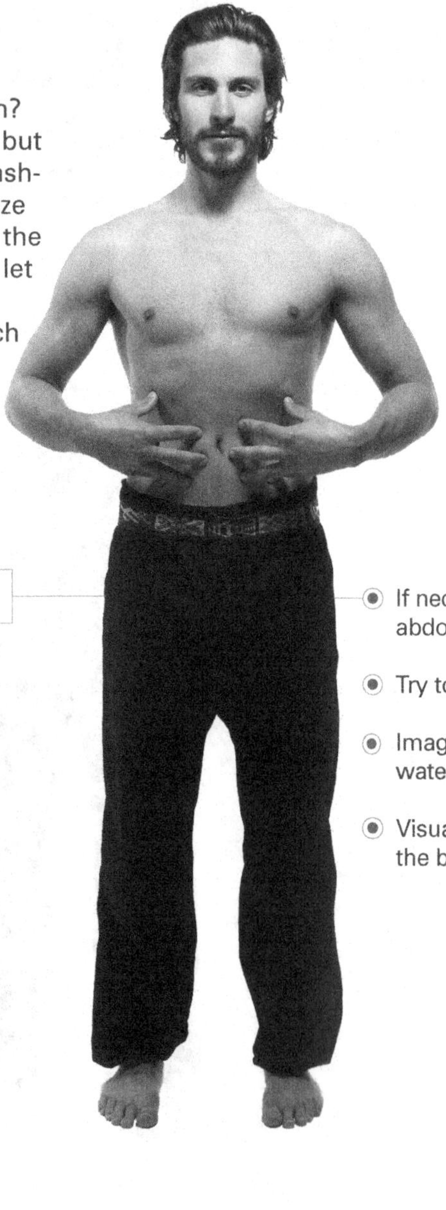

Fig. 3: Diaphragmatic Exhalation

- If necessary, cough to engage the abdominals.

- Try to squeeze out all the air.

- Imagine that you are wringing water out of a towel.

- Visualize the abs wrapping around the body's core to empty the breath.

Practice these for a minimum of ten breaths. If you lose focus, cough to reset your rhythm. It may also help to take more shallow breaths than you normally do. For example, we always say, "Take a deep breath." But that is only half the equation. The other half is breathing out.

Most people like to rest on 90 or 100 percent of their lung capacity. When they exhale, they release only 20 or 30 percent of the volume. This means the bottom of the barrel is never emptied. It's like lung constipation. It's like a cook who chops new tomatoes every day and throws them in a jar on top of the old ones. Can you imagine what that jar of tomatoes would look like? Likewise, if we don't empty out all the way, the air in our lungs becomes stale and heavy. Sure, most people could stand to lose a few pounds, but in many cases, that distension is not really a beer belly, but an air belly. When we exhale all the way, we appear to lose weight immediately.

Granted, it's a big shift, and diaphragmatic breathing takes a little getting used to, but when you begin to rest on empty, each molecule of air can be used. The exhalation serves to lengthen your spine and propel you up against the hand of gravity. The beauty of the forced exhalation is that it empties out your lungs and brings in new oxygen. As your abdominals wake up, you get free crunches every time you exhale—the muscles develop an elasticity that actually does the work for you! And then a radical transformation happens: instead of resting on full and allowing the stomach to flop over, you rest on empty, and the dynamic elasticity massages your internal organs, aligns your posture, calms the mind, and fills you with energy. Just by breathing properly.

Be warned. The D-breath is habit forming. This kind of breathing is so natural and feels so good that after just a few weeks you will be addicted.

More than any other health, fitness, or wellness program—cardio, diet plans, supplements, weight training—this one choice, this singular shift in awareness, will illuminate and assist your growth in all other directions. *Mastering the breath is the key to unlocking the power of any other exercise.* What's more, it is the only way to arrive at that permanent state of being where an abundance of life energy flows. Unlocking the diaphragm dismantles the armor that keeps our hearts in a cage.

Enjoy the magnetic buoyancy of an inspired existence.

BREATHING MEDITATION

Find a comfortable, seated position and relax your mind. Focus your awareness on your heart center or solar plexus. Then take a deep breath into your diaphragm, counting to six. Imagine that you are drawing the energy up to your third eye. Hold for three beats, imagining that you are energizing your pineal gland. Now, using your diaphragm to push the breath out, exhale for six counts. Continue breathing like this for three sets of ten, taking a brief pause to relax and breath normally between repetitions. Focus on the space between your eyebrows and feel the radiant light from your heart gathering in the brain, filling you with universal love and awareness.

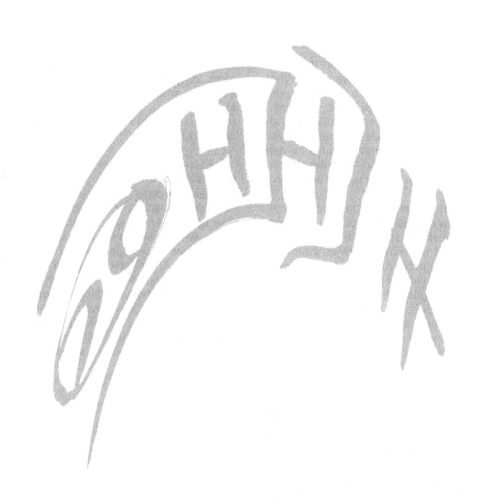

Chapter 3. *The Basic Warm-Up*

The Basic Warm-Up is based on the classic martial arts or gymnastics warm-up. Where traditionally the warm-up was a brief antecedent to practice, here it is the practice. Nothing is more effective for movement reeducation and for connecting you to the basic elements of your body than this. It is also highly valuable for gaining therapeutic information—for determining which areas of the body need special attention or treatment.

This form is adapted from the warm-up taught to me by a Cuban gymnast. He was thirty-six when we met and still performing flips with ease. I watched his movements as you would watch a jaguar. I noticed the way his abdomen was woven like a vertical snake belt, the way his shoulders would glide and explode with power, and the lean efficiency of his arms and legs.

The exercises that follow, originally done in a linear form, can also be executed using a relaxed form. In other words, instead of lots of straight lines and locked joints, you can let everything flow in circles. In doing so, the exercises systematically map, clean, and link the neuronal infrastructure; oil and lubricate every single joint; and also act like a translation dictionary, deciphering the language of the body. Each time you practice you can refine the quality of your movements.

Come to center. Take a deep breath and feel your feet on the ground. Rock forward and back to find the *weightless zone* (see chap. 1). It is important to return to this center after each and every movement. Go into the Basic Stance, send roots down, and do a few diaphragmatic breaths (D-breaths). This way, your body can integrate the information and begin to create new patterns. As you begin, keep in mind the circle of ease, the smooth and optimal range of motion for each joint. If you hear any clicks or pops, try to make the circle smaller until you find the efficiency zone.

Each of these exercises can be approached from different angles. You can hold them for ten or twenty breaths and they will function much like a yoga posture, or you can intensify the exercise by speeding it up. In general, you want to move with a moderate to fast tempo and do approximately ten repetitions of each dynamic movement. The stretches can be held for five or ten counts. The idea is to create and maintain movement pathways, which is more about conscious repetition than duration of the movement. Long-term practice of the Basic Warm-Up will prevent many postural distortions and disruptions of chi and create a strong and balanced body.

THE BASIC WARM-UP EXERCISE SET
1. Arm Circles

Reach your arms overhead and begin to do large circles on the sides of your body. Straighten the elbows, try to have as little friction as possible in the shoulder girdle, and extend the energy through the hands. Do ten reps and then reverse.

Fig. 3.1: Arm Circles

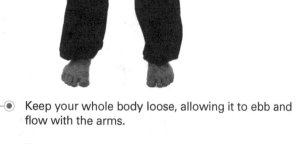

- Keep your whole body loose, allowing it to ebb and flow with the arms.

- Think of all the muscles working in a chain, like a brigade.

- Stay on a vertical axis. Try not to rock back on the heels.

2. Spinal Twists

Return to the Basic Stance and take a deep breath. Now bend your knees a little extra and let your arms fall by your sides. Rock back and forth while maintaining a vertical axis. Tuck your pelvis under slightly, but relax the hips. Focus on turning the ribcage independently of the pelvis.

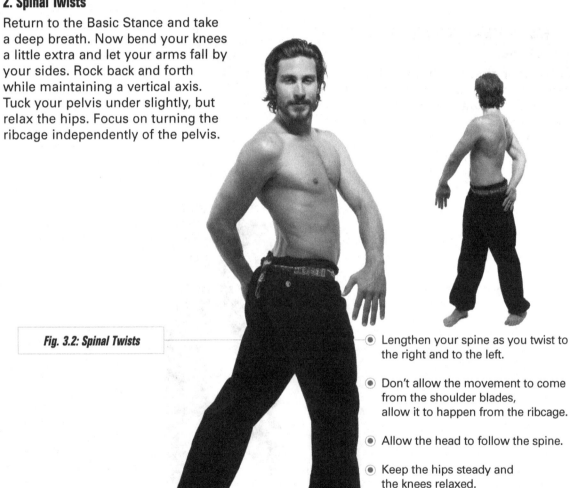

Fig. 3.2: Spinal Twists

⊙ Lengthen your spine as you twist to the right and to the left.

⊙ Don't allow the movement to come from the shoulder blades, allow it to happen from the ribcage.

⊙ Allow the head to follow the spine.

⊙ Keep the hips steady and the knees relaxed.

3. Shoulder Rolls

Return to the Basic Stance and let your hands rest at your sides. Keep your shoulders wide as you circle them backward. Think of moving through four quadrants. Begin by going back and be sure to lift all the way up, all the way back, all the way down, and all the way forward again. Repeat for ten reps, and then reverse direction.

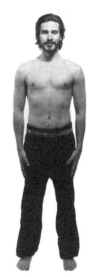

Fig. 3.3: Shoulder Rolls

- ◉ Keep the shoulders wide.

- ◉ Try to glide over the ribcage.

- ◉ Keep the spine steady.

- ◉ Move smooth.

4. Triceps Stretch

Return to center. Reach both arms over your head and bend them so that the two arms create a box. Fold one arm down behind your back and try to touch the shoulder blade on the same side. Push back gently on the elbow with the opposite hand.

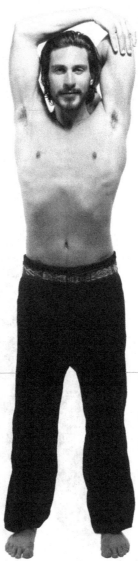

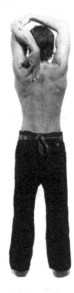

Fig. 3.4: Triceps Stretch

- ⦿ Use the lats (your back, side muscles) to stabilize the shoulders.

- ⦿ Use the abs to anchor the ribcage.

- ⦿ Don't allow the chest to rotate.

- ⦿ Keep the hips steady.

5. Deltoid Stretches

Shake out your arms and let them
rest at your sides. Then bring one
arm straight in front of you, turn it
out, palms up, and lock the elbow.
Slowly cross your body with that
arm and pull it in gently using the
opposite forearm.

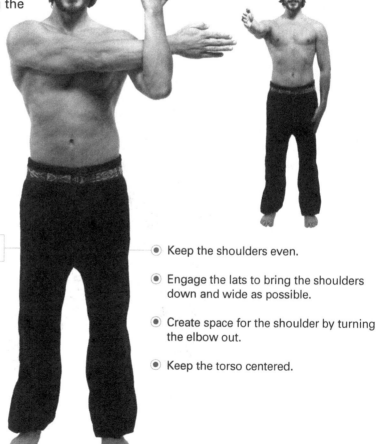

Fig. 3.5: Deltoid Stretches

- Keep the shoulders even.

- Engage the lats to bring the shoulders
  down and wide as possible.

- Create space for the shoulder by turning
  the elbow out.

- Keep the torso centered.

6. Side Stretch (from horse stance)

Return to center and feel the alignment in your entire body. Then spread your feet wide and bend your knees, dropping the energy down into your quads. This is the horse stance. Lean slightly into one leg, and reach the same arm over your head. Straighten the other leg slightly and stretch.

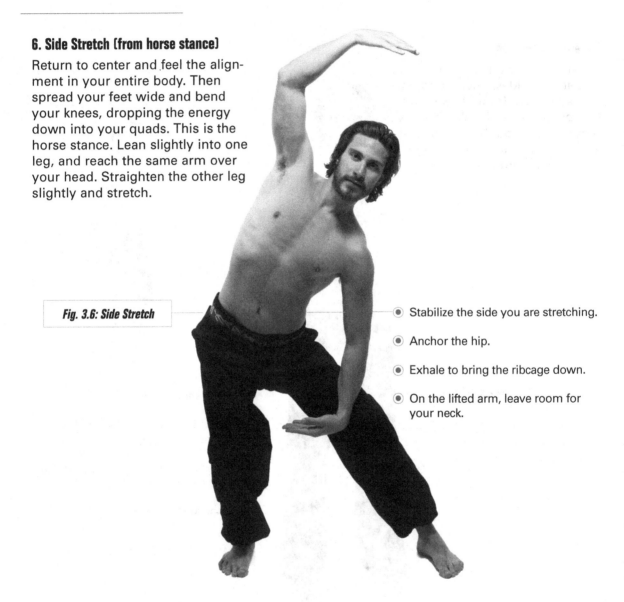

Fig. 3.6: Side Stretch

- Stabilize the side you are stretching.

- Anchor the hip.

- Exhale to bring the ribcage down.

- On the lifted arm, leave room for your neck.

7. The Fountain of Youth

Remain in horse stance and rotate left, facing your left knee so that you are in a left-lunge position. Bring your right arm up so there is one continuous line from your back foot to your right hand. Bring your left arm down and back to push gently on the straight, back leg. Try to open the hip so that the lower back does not over compress. Use your abs to support you from the front and to control the intensity of the stretch. Then in one smooth motion, swing your right arm down while rotating to the right, so that you are facing your right knee, and swing your left arm up. The arm that stretches up should always be on the same side as the leg that is back.

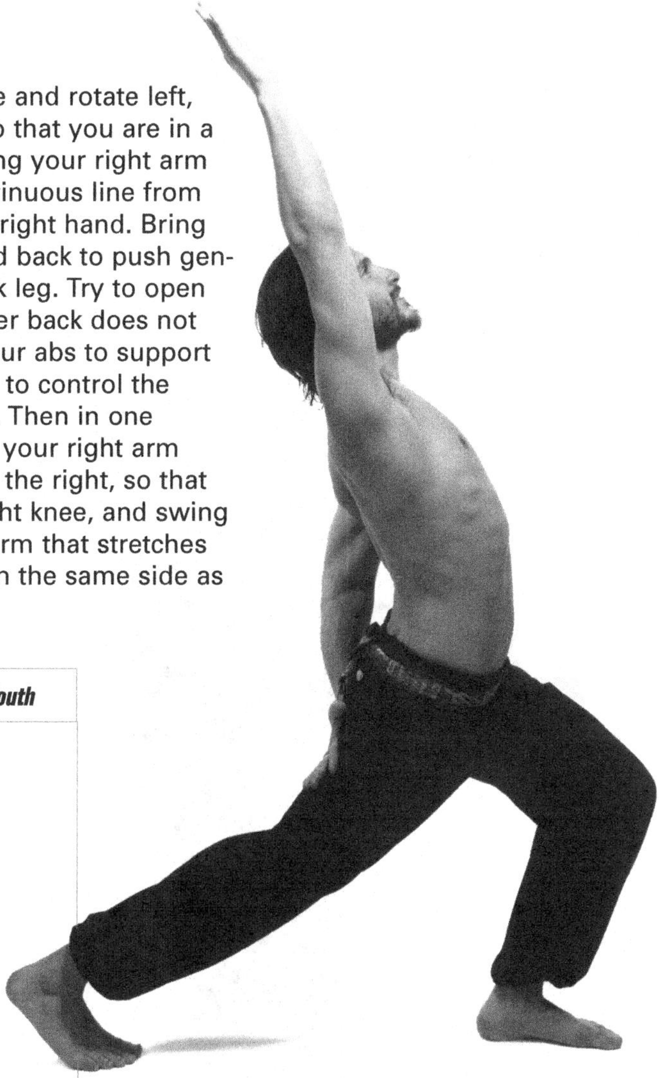

Fig. 3.7: The Fountain of Youth

- Imagine that you are a bow with an arrow resting on top of your hip.

- Try to make a continuous stretch from your feet to your hands.

- Breathe in as the arm comes up and use the abs to direct the stretch.

8. Hip Circles

Stand with your feet and knees together and place your hands on your hips. Keep your head steady and begin to circle your hips. Keep your feet planted on the ground and swivel at the knees. Circle for a count of ten to the right and then reverse direction.

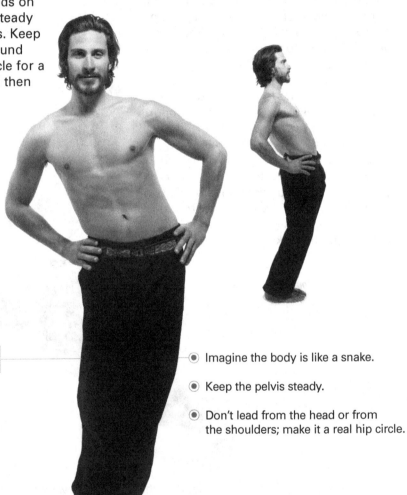

Fig. 3.8: Hip Circles

◉ Imagine the body is like a snake.

◉ Keep the pelvis steady.

◉ Don't lead from the head or from the shoulders; make it a real hip circle.

9. Knee Circles

Shake out your legs and stand with your feet together and knees touching. Bend at the waist, with your knees slightly bent, and place your hands on your knees. Lift your spine and circle your knees for a count of ten in both directions.

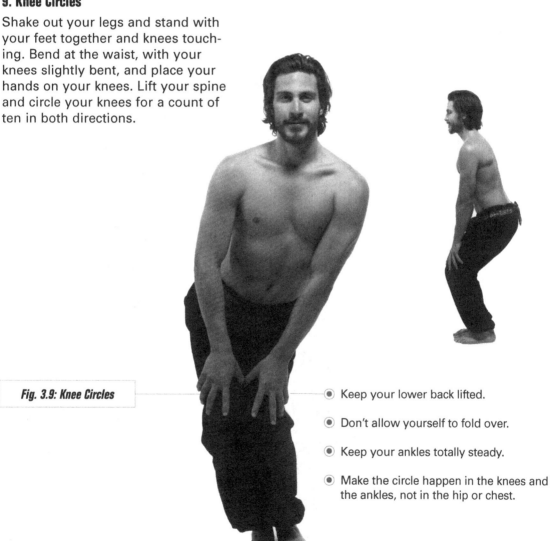

Fig. 3.9: Knee Circles

- Keep your lower back lifted.

- Don't allow yourself to fold over.

- Keep your ankles totally steady.

- Make the circle happen in the knees and the ankles, not in the hip or chest.

10. Elbow Circles

Stand with the feet shoulder-width apart. Lift your right arm chest-high and rest your elbow in the opposite hand. Then circle the forearm from the elbow. Try to feel the circle of ease, the point of least resistance. Circle to the left for a count of ten and then to the right. Switch to your left arm and repeat.

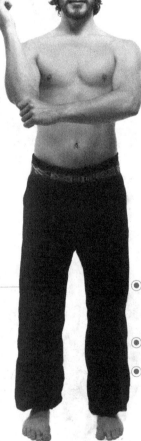
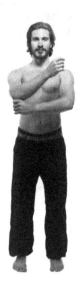

Fig. 3.10: Elbow Circles

- Keep your elbow steady and allow only the forearm to move in a circle as the upper arm remains still, only rotating internally.

- Try to have a smooth relaxed motion.

- Keep the rest of the body planted.

11. Upward Wrist Stretch

Lower your arms and shake them out. Rest. Place one hand in front with the palm up. Use the other hand to gently pull down and stretch the underside of the wrist. This will help to loosen the carpal tunnel. Try not to twist the hand too much, but to stretch all the lines equally. Switch hands.

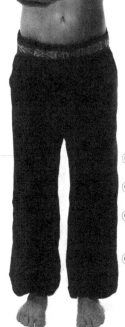
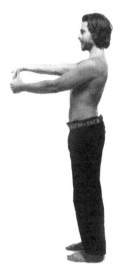

Fig. 3.11: Upward Wrist Stretch

- Don't allow your elbows to rotate in or out.

- Be aware of your shoulders' alignment.

- Try to feel the stretch not only in the wrist, but also all the way up to the forearm.

- Relax the opposing muscles.

12. Downward Wrist Stretch

Turn your hand over so the palm is down. Straighten the elbow. Pull your hand toward the chest with the opposite hand and stretch the top of the forearm.

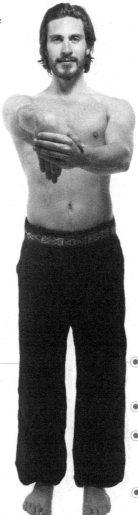
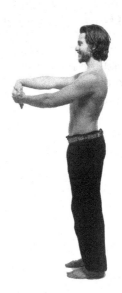

Fig. 3.12: Downward Wrist Stretch

- Rotate your elbow up to get maximal stretch.

- Keep your back straight.

- Wrap your hand over the top of the hand you are stretching and not just over the fingers.

- Feel your arm connect to your core strength.

13. Lateral Neck Stretches

Bring your feet shoulder-width apart and let your arms rest at their sides. Stretch your arms down and hands out, and curl the fingers up to anchor your shoulder blades. Stretch your head from side to side, then forward and back. When you stretch, make sure to lift all the way up before going over so that you can have maximal extension.

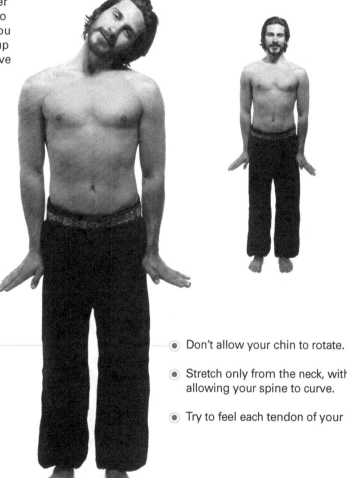

Fig. 3.13: Lateral Neck Stretches

⊙ Don't allow your chin to rotate.

⊙ Stretch only from the neck, without allowing your spine to curve.

⊙ Try to feel each tendon of your neck.

14. Forward-and-Back Neck Stretch

Return to center and pull your head up toward the sky, lengthening your cervical vertebrae. Then slowly fold down, bringing your chin to your chest. Lift up and slowly stretch back, making sure to open your throat and the upper part of your sternum.

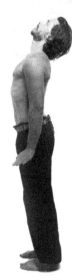

Fig. 3.14: Forward-and-Back Neck Stretch

⊙ Keeping your spine steady, feel the space between each of your vertebrae.

⊙ When you arch back, lift up first and don't hyperextend your neck.

⊙ Be sure to open your chest to the sky.

⊙ Feel the muscles of your neck unsticking.

15. Ankle Stretches

This exercise is very important for balance, articulation, and circulation. Stand on one leg, bend at the knee, and lift the other leg a few inches off of the ground. Keeping your hip steady, point and flex your lifted foot ten times. Following that, circle your ankle around in each direction ten times, making sure that the circles are smooth and symmetrical. Repeat on the other side.

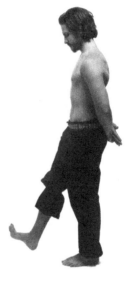

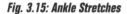

Fig. 3.15: Ankle Stretches

⦿ Keep the rest of your leg steady.

⦿ Find the optimal range of motion.

⦿ Relax your toes.

⦿ Keep your upper body lifted.

⦿ Keep space in the joint;
no clicks and pops.

16. Knee Orbits

Lift one leg and let your foot hang.
Keep your knee steady and allow
only your upper leg to rotate in and
out as you trace circles above the
floor with the foot.

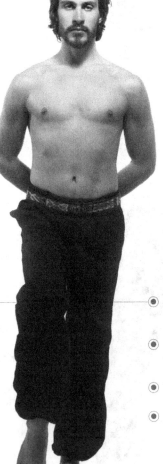

Fig. 3.16: Knee Orbits

◉ Isolate the movement so your upper leg
is rotating but not lifting or lowering.

◉ Make sure your lower back is lifted and
your standing leg steady.

◉ Try to make a smooth 360-degree circle.

◉ Don't over grip the floor; keep your toes
relaxed on your standing leg.

17. Quad Stretch

Keeping the quads open is one of the keys to avoiding hip replacements and maintaining overall vitality. Often people stretch only the lower part of the muscle and fail to open the crux of the hip. In order to get the maximum benefit from the stretch, it is important to recruit the muscles in the abdomen to stabilize the pelvis. Stand on one leg and grab the opposite foot behind you with your hand. Push forward from the hip so there is a straight line from the chest to the knee.

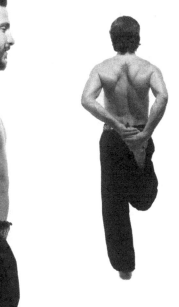

Fig. 3.17: Quad Stretch

⦿ Think of the body as a bow, with the arrow resting on the hip.

⦿ Stretch the origin of the quads.

⦿ Lift up through the top of the head.

⦿ Keep the lower back extended.

18. The Swoop

Stand with your feet shoulder-width apart and your knees slightly bent. Reach your arms over your head and lengthen your spine. Roll down one vertebra at a time until your hands brush the floor. Keep your neck relaxed and your arms overhead. Then, with a flat back, extend your shoulders out as you come up, keeping your elbows slightly behind your ears. As you become more comfortable with this exercise, you can straighten your legs and try for maximal spinal extension.

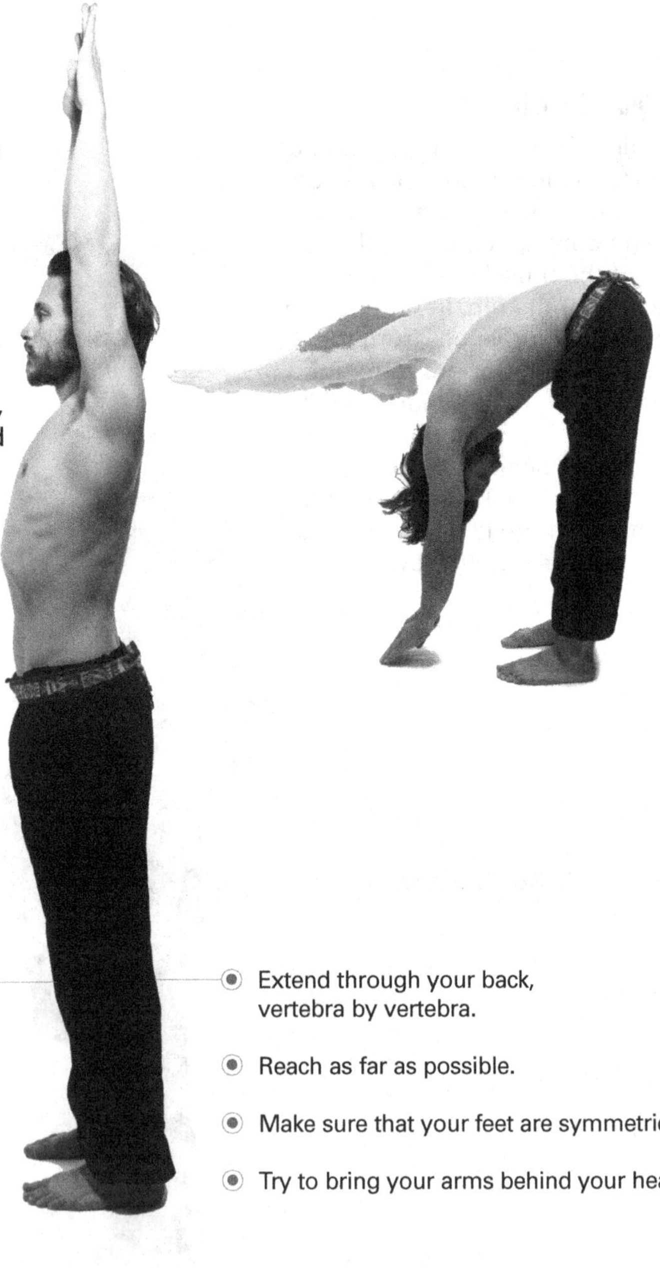

Fig. 3.18: The Swoop

- Extend through your back, vertebra by vertebra.

- Reach as far as possible.

- Make sure that your feet are symmetrical.

- Try to bring your arms behind your head.

THE CHILL LIST. *Formulating a Personal Checklist*

In essence, these exercises are about ease—the idea is to find it as often as possible and stay there as long as possible. The following tips are things to keep in mind as you go through the Basic Warm-Up and as you continue with the program. Each of us has our own personal challenges. In the beginning, we may need to constantly remind ourselves of the ways that we lose our center, but with affirmation comes change, and with patience and practice comes accomplishment.

The notes listed below are very common reminders, and some are likely to be applicable to your body. These are the corrections I have made with countless clients. Try not to get hung up on "mistakes," but at the same time be strict with yourself as you look for your center. You will find that simple movements that are "easy" when you are not *present** become extremely effective when you show up. With this check list, checking in with yourself from time to time, not just when exercising, will increase your ability to *chill* all day long.

Try not to lean back on your heels.
Keep your weight evenly distributed over the three points of your foot—the heel and the two lateral aspects of the ball.

Try not to lean back on your back.
Muscles pull much better than they push. If I want to do a biceps curl, it is the biceps that pull the weight up, not the triceps pushing. Likewise, a synergistic balance between the abdominal muscles and the back should maintain posture, but all too often, we rely on our back muscles, and they end up, sometimes begrudgingly, holding us up all day.

Relax your buttocks.
This is one of the tricks in relaxing the back: your buttocks and your lower back are synergistic, so if you can relax the glutes, which is easy to accomplish, then you can often release the lower back as well.

Engage the abdominals.
Sometimes opposition is the key to balance. It can be difficult to relax your back, but by engaging our abdominals, we can often balance out the tension. This is the concept of yin and yang—turning one on turns the other off.

Drop the weight into your quads.
Whenever we are out of alignment, tension builds up. To reduce tension in your back, drop some of the tension into your quads. They are the natural weight-bearing group, and they distribute the energy right down to the ground.

Bend your knees slightly.
This is another aspect of dropping the weight back down to the earth and of not interrupting the flow of gravity. The slight bend in your knee opens the floodgates.

Tuck your pelvis.
A slight tuck of the pelvis allows the waves of your body to flow in a natural rhythm. If you do all the other components of the checklist, your pelvis will most likely tuck on its own. If not, rotate it forward a little bit—this is the opposite movement of sticking your buttocks out.

Paying attention with your full awareness—sensory, mental, emotional.

Lengthen your neck.

Spinal power comes from all the vertebrae working like a spring. Unfortunately, some or many of the coils are often locked together. Real back extension happens when the whole spine lengthens back, but usually it is just the neck that hyperextends. To counter this, think of lifting all the way up before you go back. In this way, the spine will move through zero before going into the negative numbers (extension).

Relax your face.

Your face is a microcosm of the rest of your body, including the internal muscles. By relaxing your face, you can often become aware of other movement patterns that are detracting from the efficiency of an action, in the moment.

Drop your shoulders.

This one is ongoing. Keep checking in and relaxing your shoulders. For some reason, they love to live up by the ears.

Relax your toes.

Toes are there for balance, no doubt, but ideally, they are there only in balance emergencies. When all the other aspects are aligned, we can rest in the circle of ease—very little struggle is necessary for balance.

As you learn the Basic Warm-Up, try to continuously refine the quality of your movements. Don't just go through the motions, carefully observe, feel, and listen to your body. You must put your awareness in the driver's seat in order to unlock the potency of these exercises. Be relaxed, but put forth continuous effort. In this way, you will progress safely and swiftly.

PART II

THE MAINTENANCE SET:
EXERCISES FOR EASE

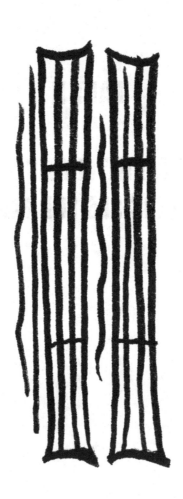

The techniques in *Weightlessness* are meant to do much more than perfect your physique. The exercises are designed to enhance self-awareness and guide us along a path of realization, toward the optimization of human potential, and to a full experience of living. Awareness, consciousness, bliss.

The Maintenance Set is a group of exercises that can be done on a daily basis. In fact, this became my daily practice in the jungle. Once you are proficient, each of the following sets will take only ten to fifteen minutes to complete and be enough to sustain a certain level of fitness. All are gentle, yet you will see profound results. This group of exercises is all you need to take on the world and stay limber for life.

These three sets can also be practiced together—as one complete workout—or separately. I suggest you wake up and do the Eight Brocades (chap. 4). In the afternoon, take a little break and do the Swimming Dragon (chap. 6). At night, before you go to sleep, do a few Sun Salutes (chap. 5), and then lie on your back and rest. You will find these exercises ease stress and flood the body with a feeling of well-being; they build strength without overdeveloping the body or creating tension. And they calm and center the human bioelectrical system, allowing us to reside in a state of ease.

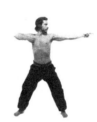

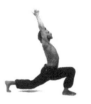

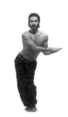

Chapter 4. *The Eight Brocades*

Chi kung literally means *working with energy* and is an ancient Chinese tradition that includes meditation, breathing, massage, and the martial arts. Because it was such an inclusive discipline—physical, poetic, artistic, metaphysical—different individuals have offered different sequences and continue to do so even today.* I learned the sequence Eight Brocades many years ago and have adapted it to my own body, making adjustments with regard to style and order. Veteran practitioners will notice a slightly different set from the traditional one—easier to learn but still highly efficient. The exercises of this form were originally introduced to maintain fitness in men exposed to extreme conditions. The set was designed to transform rigid muscles into woven, silk-like braids.

When the chi flow is smooth, we experience healthy skin and radiant health. When it is interrupted, the body's defenses are weaker, which can result in disease. There are many claims of chi kung curing disease. Although some dispute the claims, it is certainly a profound preventative medicine. It is multileveled—electrical, physical, neurological—and therefore can deeply affect the human being. Chi kung is a complete system, designed to accompany Chinese medicine.

This set is just one of many forms of chi kung that have been passed down through the years. Within each, there are many variations. If I am feeling the stress of the day or if I am thinking too much, feeling stiff, or worried, I run through the Eight Brocades and stress seems to vanish. This in itself is enough to keep you feeling good and to maintain functional strength and flexibility. If you are sick, it can begin to restore your vitality. It is gentle enough to do first thing in the morning and relaxing enough to do at night. These exercises also help the organs to function properly and align the meridian system. The Eight Brocades is also an excellent warm-up.

While practicing, try to cultivate a feeling of peace and serenity: breathe deeply and visualize the cosmic life force rejuvenating your cells. Chi kung evolved in the Buddhist and Taoist traditions where you learn to become like water; that is, to flow effortlessly past and around obstacles. In this way, the movements, which at first glance may appear simple or easy, gradually reveal how to use your body in the most graceful ways. The exercises will teach physical efficiency and minimize antagonistic tensions in the joints.

Each exercise can be done six to eight times, with some exceptions that are better kept at ten. Use your mind and your breath to direct the chi and bring awareness to your internal organs. Always open and close the form with a moment of silent meditation—to gather your energy and center your being.

---

*This classic form of chi kung has been adapted according to the principles of Integrated Exercise and therefore may differ slightly from more orthodox approaches. It is not my intention to present the traditional method.

THE EIGHT BROCADES EXERCISE SET

1. Lifting the Hands

Return to the Basic Stance and take a few diaphragmatic breaths. Try to feel your body rooting into the ground. Lace the fingers together and rest the knuckles on the top of your head. On inhalation, lift the arms straight up to the sky, and then lower them down on exhalation. After six reps, turn the hands over and continue; this time the palms will be resting on the head.

Fig. 4.1a: Lifting the Hands [knuckles down]

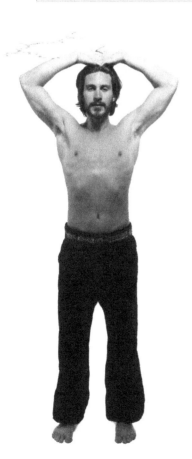
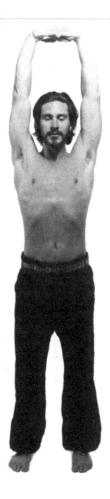

- Use your breath to anchor the ribcage.

- Continue to reach up and back as much as possible as you lift your arms.

- Look up occasionally to make sure your arms are symmetrical.

- Try to leave space between your shoulders and your neck.

Fig. 4.1b: Lifting the Hands [palms down]

- ◉ Continue to breathe as you lift your arms.
- ◉ Keep your shoulders down.
- ◉ Let your weight drop down into the earth.
- ◉ Try to move with maximum efficiency.

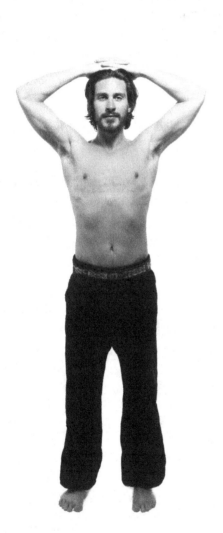
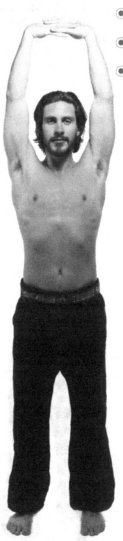

2. Rolling Down to Create an Elastic Spine

True spinal health is achieved when we expand the space between each
vertebra. Stand in the Basic Stance and place your hands on the backs of
your legs, so they are cupping the buttocks. Inhale as you roll down one
vertebra at a time into a forward bend, simultaneously sliding your arms
down the backs of your legs. Do not flop over; instead imagine that you are
a bow, with the coil and stretch of bamboo. Then roll back up. When you
are standing straight, lift your heels and balance on your toes. Repeat six to
eight times.

Fig. 4.2: Elastic Spine

- Expand the space between each of your vertebra.

- Use your breath to stretch.

- When you lift your heels, be careful not to roll out; keep the alignment in your ankle.

- Push straight up with your head.

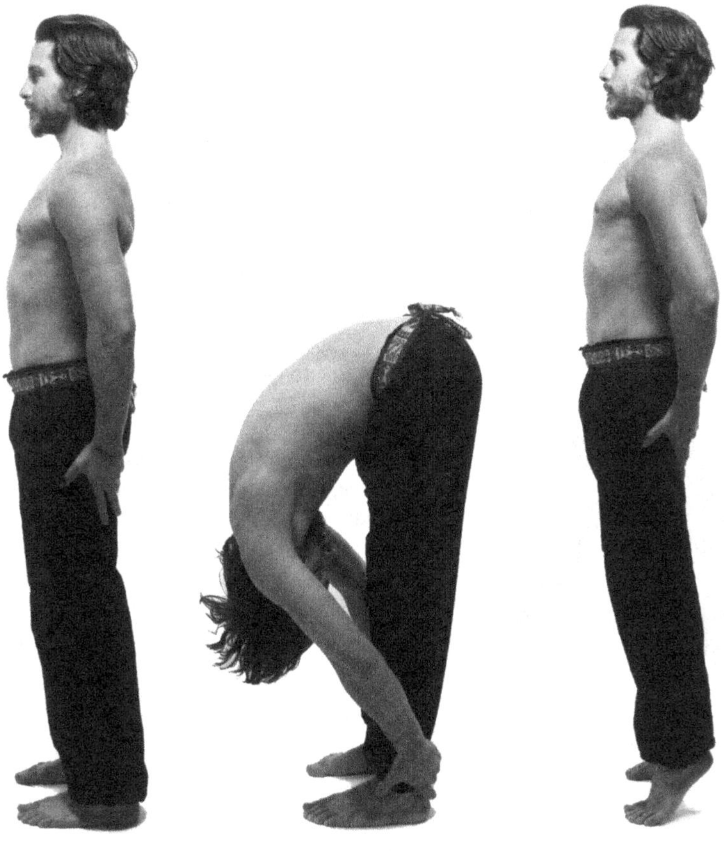

3. Drawing the Bow

Return to center and spread your legs considerably wider, but do not allow your feet to turn out excessively—legs should be symmetrical. Drop your weight into your quads and lift up out of your spine. This is the horse stance. Now, bring both hands in front of you with the palms facing the chest. On inhalation, extend one arm out and coil the other one as if you are drawing a bow. Hold for a breath and then bring your hands back in front with the same energy—without "shooting the arrow"—then repeat.

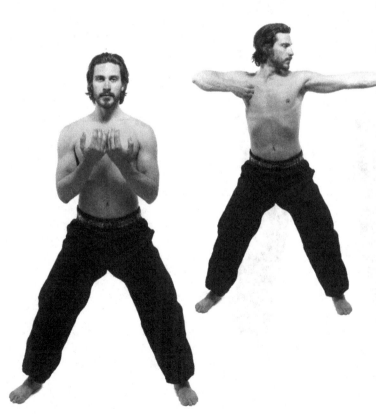

Fig 4.3: Drawing the Bow

- The hand holding the bow should be filled with energy.

- The hand holding the string should be shoulder height.

- Keep your weight evenly centered over your legs.

- Imagine an elastic band between your two hands.

- Return to center between each repetition.

- Don't allow the shoulders to break back, open them wide from the blades.

4. Spinal Rotation

Return to the horse stance and place your hands on your knees. Tuck your belly and lengthen as much as possible out of your spine. Take a deep breath in, and on exhalation, rotate to one side. Return to center. Repeat in both directions six to eight times. When you are familiar with this movement, rotate again, and this time lower the chest to one leg and swoop around so you end up with your chest on the opposite leg. Then return to center. Repeat in both directions.

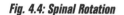

Fig. 4.4: Spinal Rotation

- Use your arms to stabilize your hips, but don't let the hips rotate—only the spine should turn.

- Try to center your movement in your lower back. Don't over-twist in the shoulders.

- Don't lead with the head; allow it to complete the movement.

- Focus on unsticking your ribcage from the pelvis.

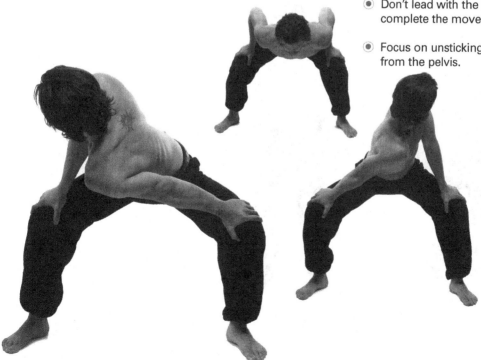

5. Stretching the Neck with the Breath

Bring your feet back to shoulder-width apart and allow your arms to fall by your sides. Curl your fingers up and extend them out. As you inhale, lift your heels and rotate your head to one side. Lower your heels and return to center. Lift and rotate to the other side. After you have done ten rotations on each side, bring your hands to kidney level and, with fingers facing down, run the whole set again (variation B). Then cup the buttocks and repeat the exercise with hands in that position, rotating to the left and to the right ten times (variation C). The different hand positions will stretch different meridians, and the repetition will give you an effective calf workout.

| Fig. 4.5a: Stretching the Neck |

⊙ Make sure your feet are aligned as you lift.

⊙ Don't allow your spine to rotate; only turn your neck.

⊙ Lift first and then turn.

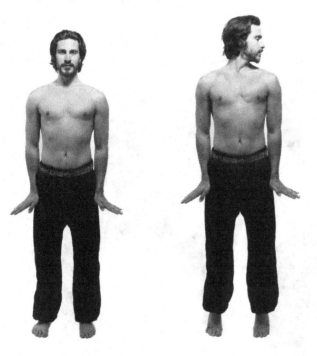

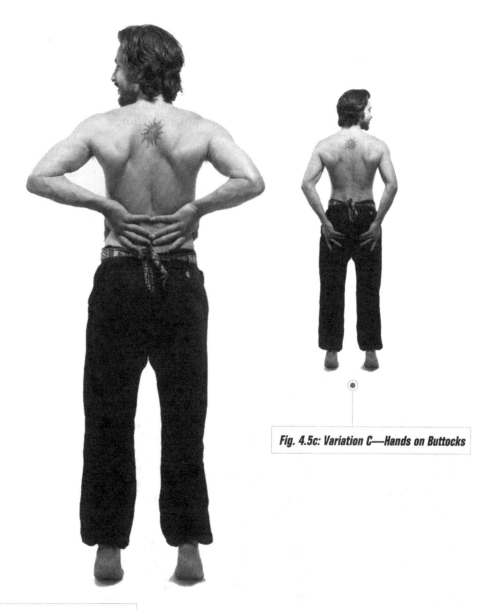

Fig. 4.5c: Variation C—Hands on Buttocks

Fig. 4.5b: Variation B—Hands on Kidneys

6. The Windmill

Return to the Basic Stance and bring your arms in front of you, elbows out, hands waist-high with fingertips touching. With your palms out, push your right hand away and up over your head, and your left one down—as if stretching a rubber band between them. Lift your hand without overusing the pectorals or neck muscles, and with considerable external rotation (turning out). You should feel a stretch in your lower hand as you push down. Reverse the movement to return to center and switch arms, moving your left hand away and up and your right hand down. Repeat full two-sided movement eight times.

Fig. 4.6a: The Windmill (front)

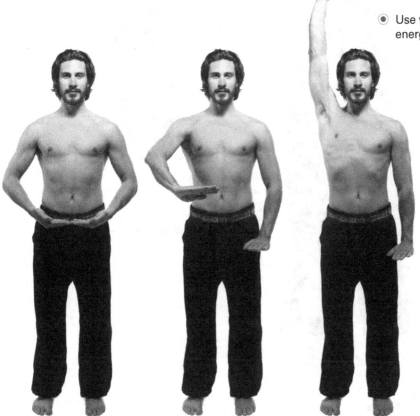

- Allow your shoulder blades to rotate back.

- Keep your hands somewhat relaxed.

- Use your intention to direct the energy out, up, and down.

Windmill Variation

To exercise the lateral rotation of the shoulder blades, you can do a similar exercise behind your back. Reach one arm behind you and up and the other behind you and down—as if you are trying to touch your hands behind your back, but continue to move. Then, keeping the elbows steady, straighten the arms in a figure eight movement. Rotate your straightened arms around to the other side and repeat for a total of ten reps.

Fig. 4.6b: Windmill Variation B (back)

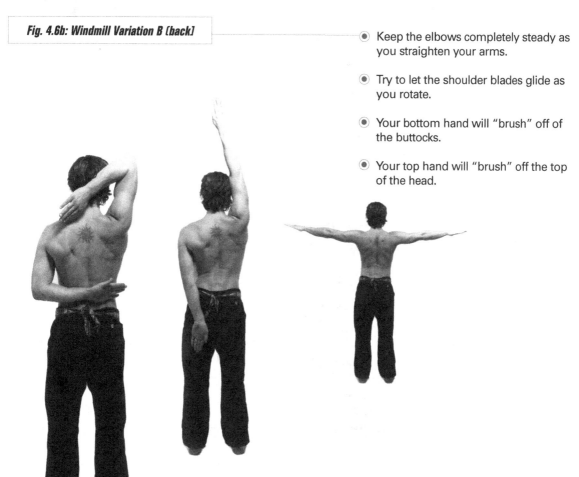

- Keep the elbows completely steady as you straighten your arms.

- Try to let the shoulder blades glide as you rotate.

- Your bottom hand will "brush" off of the buttocks.

- Your top hand will "brush" off the top of the head.

7. Punching from the Hip

This is another exercise designed to help unstick the pelvis from the ribcage, and it also teaches you to connect your abs to the power of the breath. Stand in the horse stance and make fists with your hands resting at your hips. Focus your eyes forward, and as you exhale, punch forward without stressing your shoulder joint. Try to get maximal twist out of your abdomen.

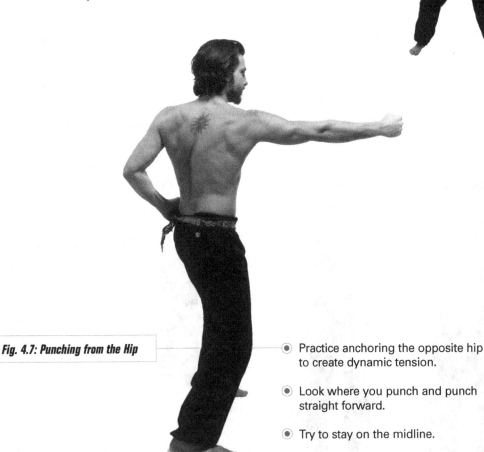

Fig. 4.7: Punching from the Hip

- Practice anchoring the opposite hip to create dynamic tension.

- Look where you punch and punch straight forward.

- Try to stay on the midline.

8. Swooping

Stand with your feet slightly more than shoulder-width apart and clasp your hands together over your head. Fold down into a forward bend. As you lift up, lead with your arms so that you are arching back and getting full extension from the shoulder blades. The swoop should be done in one smooth motion.

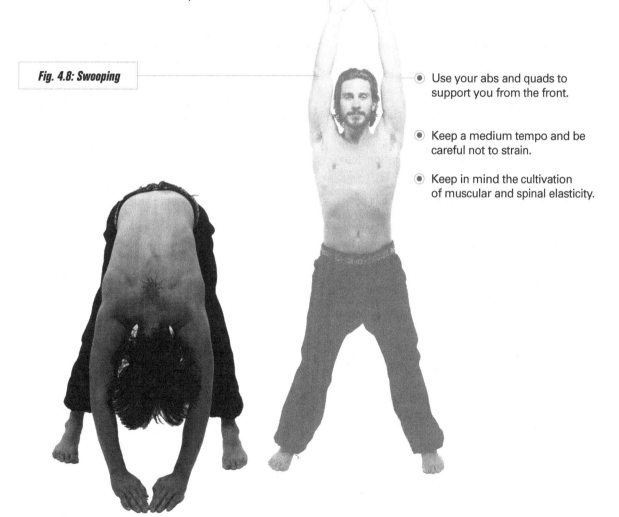

Fig. 4.8: Swooping

- Use your abs and quads to support you from the front.

- Keep a medium tempo and be careful not to strain.

- Keep in mind the cultivation of muscular and spinal elasticity.

THE EFFICIENCY ZONE

The following are guidelines for an efficient practice.
These are meta-principles equally applicable to exercise and to life.

1. You need to minimize antagonistic tension. Use only the necessary amount of energy. In other words, moving an object should only take x amount of force. However, if you have antagonistic tension, it takes x plus whatever drag the opposing muscle group provides. The state of antagonistic tension compounds the physical reality and multiplies the effects of age, weight, and stress. Efficiency reduces this equation, leaving you with a feeling of weightlessness.

2. Synergistic curves lead to optimal full body power. When all the different joints work together and are connected in the Basic Stance, you tap into an explosiveness that is exponentially greater than that of disintegrated strength. Imagine a weightlifter: his bicep may be stronger than the bicep of a person doing Integrated Exercise, but when it comes to the application of force, power is determined not just by that bicep but also by the combination of other joints and levers.

3. Sustain minimal flexibility. If a joint can't move into a position, then its power will be compromised and it may default into an unsuitable position or action. By sustaining flexibility, you can position the moving limb for maximal efficiency and effectiveness.

4. Sustain minimal strength. Muscles should have enough power to perform daily tasks, but if they are atrophied or deficient, corresponding groups may have to overwork. You want to recruit the right muscle groups for the given action. If all muscles are functional, then it isn't necessary for any of your muscle groups to default.

5. Coordinate breath with action. Use the power of the breath to direct the activity. Generally, use a forced exhalation whenever you are exerting force. In this way, the mind leads the chi.

6. No swervy head. There is a saying: "When sitting, just sit; when walking, just walk; above all, don't wobble." To move efficiently, you must be in the present moment. If your mind is somewhere else, your body will be on automatic pilot and resort to instinctual patterns rather than conscious ease. *You have got to be present.* Control your eyes, control your breath, and release your mind.

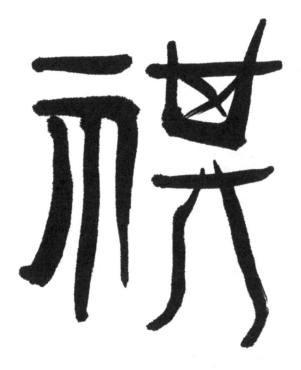

Chapter 5. *The Sun Salute*

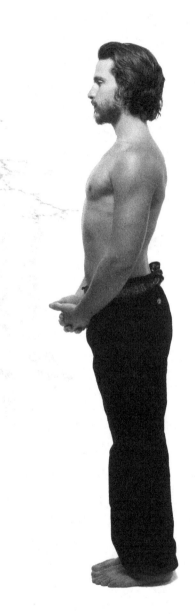

The Sun Salute is a classic sequence in many schools of yoga. In keeping with the principles of Integrated Exercise, there are many different ways to approach this form. You can hold each posture for three, five, or more breaths. Or you can flow through the entire motion, almost like dance. Sometimes people go as fast as they can.

This adaptation is designed to be relatively easy, safe, and suitable to complete every day. These exercises alone are sufficient to keep the body strong and limber. It is especially useful for opening up the quadriceps, stretching the spine, and giving flexibility to the backs of the legs. If you like, you can do a few push-ups after the plank position to add a strength-building element to the Sun Salute.

It is important for all of us to find the discipline to be your own teacher and develop a personal practice. Search for the voice in your head that will keep you motivated. Someone once said, "Isn't exercise sadomasochistic?" and the guru answered, "Only exercise without awareness." If you are going through the motions but not actually mentally present, then you are in essence torturing yourself, and there is little reason for the exercise. Whereas if you really show up, you may suffer more in the moment, but you will reap 100 percent of the benefit.

In other words, try to maintain complete awareness through all the postures, from the beginning to the end. Exhale fully, extend through the joints, keep your eyes focused, and try to move gracefully. These are movements that will keep you connected to life.

THE SUN SALUTE FORM IN TEN MOVEMENTS
1. Back Bend (back extension)

Stand with your feet shoulder-width apart and lace your fingers together in front of you. Reach your clasped hands over your head, lengthening your spine upward, and then lean back, making sure to use your abdominals and quads to support your back. Remember, muscles pull much better than they push. In other words, don't let your lower back hold you up by working it like a wedge; instead, support yourself from the front of the body and push your pelvis all the way forward.

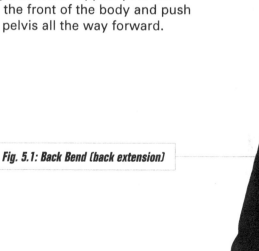
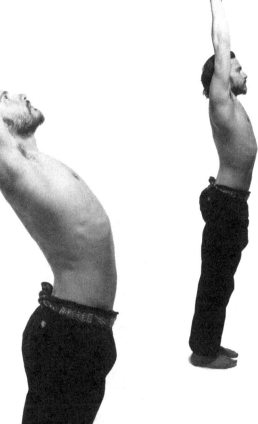

| Fig. 5.1: Back Bend (back extension) |

- Inhale.

- Be sure to lift up first. Stretch your shoulders open.

- Don't allow your neck to hyperextend.

- Use your breath to contract your ribs. Stretch your shoulders open.

2. Forward Bend

Slowly fold forward, letting your hands go, and reach for your toes. Flex your buttocks, keeping your knees slightly bent. Slowly bring your head toward your shins and stretch. If you like, you can grab behind your ankles to hold the stretch. Bend and straighten your knees* several times —slowly and gently; don't bounce.

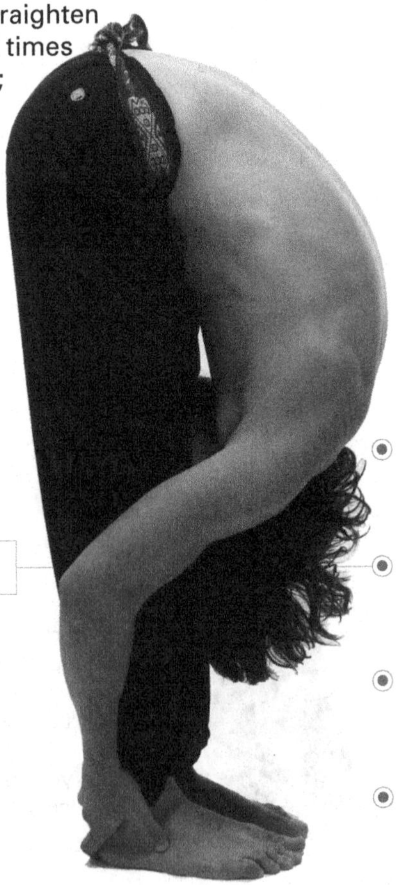

Fig. 5.2: Forward Bend

- Exhale. In order to create maximum length in your lower back, lift up and out of your pelvis.

- Focus the stretch on your upper hamstrings, and also on the sacroiliac joint, where your sacrum attaches to your pelvis.

- Don't allow yourself to back off as you exhale. Instead, use every part of each breath to advance your stretch.

- When you have improved your flexibility, you can work on straightening your knees.

There is a lot of discussion about whether or not to straighten the knees. If you get deeper into yoga, there will come a point where it will be necessary. But it is of the utmost importance that, when straightening the knees, you engage the quadriceps muscles; this will stabilize and protect the joint from hyperextension.

3. Lunge One

Bend your knees enough to place both hands flat on the mat or floor, shoulder-width apart. Move your right leg between your hands, and then shoot it back into a deep lunge, lowering the knee. Raise your torso to upright position, shifting your weight to balance. Arch your back to stretch your right quad. Or you can leave your hands down.

Fig. 5.3: Lunge One

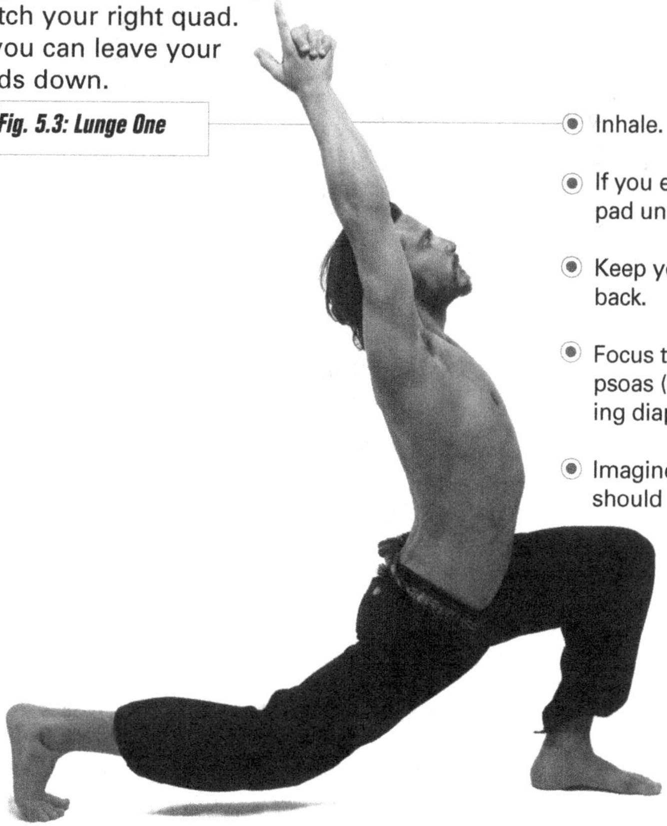

- Inhale.

- If you encounter any pain, add an extra pad under your knee.

- Keep your abs engaged to protect your back.

- Focus the stretch on your upper quad and psoas (deep abdominal muscle connecting diaphragm to hip).

- Imagine that you are a bow. The arrow should be resting just above your hip.

4. Plank Position

Bring your hands back to the floor
and shoot your left leg back, next to
your right (like a push-up position).
Rock forward, using your shoulders
as an axis, until your hands are
directly below your shoulders on the
floor. Hold. (If you like, you can mix
in 3–10 push-ups from here, before
moving to the next position. But be
sure to breathe.)

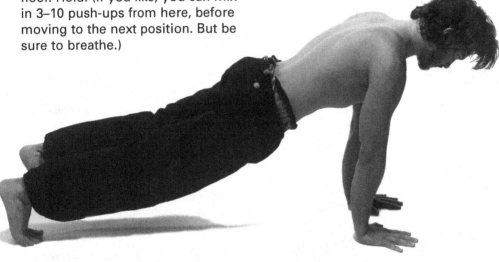

Fig. 5.4: Plank Position

⊚ Hold breath (unless doing push-ups).

⊚ Try to recruit your abs into holding you up from
   underneath.

⊚ Don't let your back sag.

⊚ Keep your buttocks tight.

⊚ Don't over use your pectorals (chest muscles).

⊚ Work on elongating your spine by pushing out
   through your feet and your head simultaneously.

5. Upward Facing Dog

Lower your chin, chest and knees to the floor and keep your elbows at your sides. (Advanced students can keep chin, chest and knees off the floor). Lay your feet flat and then arch up so that your pelvis is down but your head and back are stretching backward and upward.

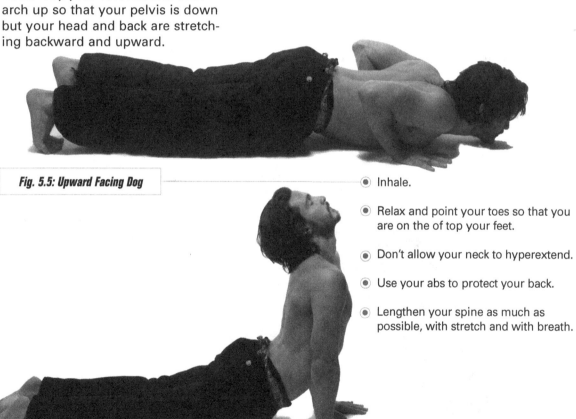

Fig. 5.5: Upward Facing Dog

- Inhale.

- Relax and point your toes so that you are on the of top your feet.

- Don't allow your neck to hyperextend.

- Use your abs to protect your back.

- Lengthen your spine as much as possible, with stretch and with breath.

6. Downward Dog

Roll over your toes so that you are on the soles of your feet. Lift your buttocks into the air, keeping your arms and legs straight, to form a triangle pose. Push your energy down through your heels and relax your head. Alternately, you may bend your knees a bit and bounce in the shoulders to open up the upper back and chest.

Fig. 5.6: Downward Dog

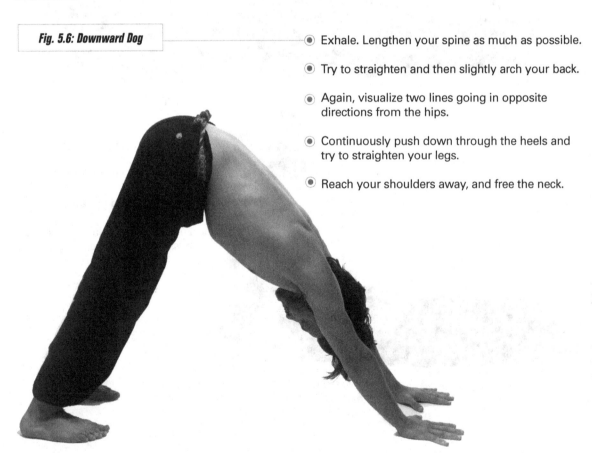

- Exhale. Lengthen your spine as much as possible.

- Try to straighten and then slightly arch your back.

- Again, visualize two lines going in opposite directions from the hips.

- Continuously push down through the heels and try to straighten your legs.

- Reach your shoulders away, and free the neck.

7. Lunge Two

At this point, you have a choice of transitions: you can move your right leg into the center and go into the lunge on the opposite side as before, or lift it straight up and stretch it to the sky before swinging it forward. Either way, bring your right foot up between your hands, keeping your left leg back. Lower your left knee and arch up as before.

- Inhale.

- Feel the elasticity through your spine and your entire body.

- Focus the stretch on the top of your hip.

- Lift your knee for more stretch.

- Use your abs to control the volume, or intensity, of the stretch.

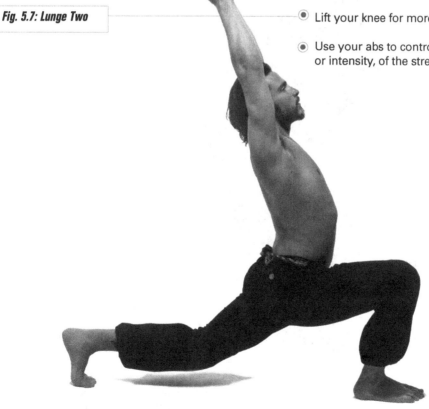

Fig. 5.7: Lunge Two

8. Forward Bend

Slowly come out of the lunge and
bring the left leg up between the
hands so that the feet are aligned.
Stretch forward again.

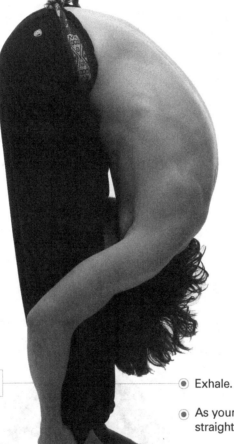

Fig. 5.8: Forward Bend

◉ Exhale.

◉ As your flexibility increases, try to
straighten the legs and the knees.

◉ Be aware of your spine and pelvis and
try to feel the back move from the very
bottom.

◉ Instead of bringing the head to the knees,
try to reach the forehead to the shins.

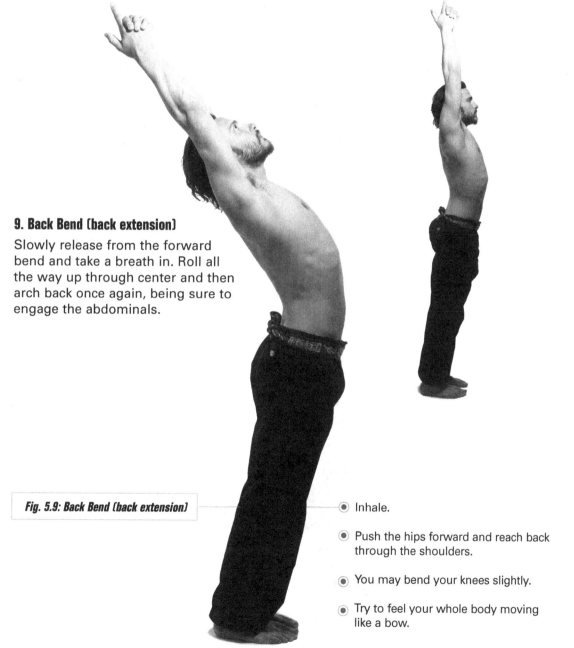

9. Back Bend (back extension)

Slowly release from the forward bend and take a breath in. Roll all the way up through center and then arch back once again, being sure to engage the abdominals.

Fig. 5.9: Back Bend (back extension)

- Inhale.

- Push the hips forward and reach back through the shoulders.

- You may bend your knees slightly.

- Try to feel your whole body moving like a bow.

10. Basic Stance

Exhale and return to the Basic Stance. Or you can keep your hands in prayer pose. Either way, take a breath, clasp hands, and get ready to repeat the series. Often it is done four times, twice in each direction.

THE SUN SALUTE can be practiced a minimum of two times, or as many as you like. This is an excellent warm-up before practicing exercises from the Advancement Set. It is also good preparation before meditating. You will notice that by the fourth set you are considerably more flexible. If the exercises become part of your daily life and you continue them over the long term, you will maintain agility and power, and prevent most disturbances in your field of energy.

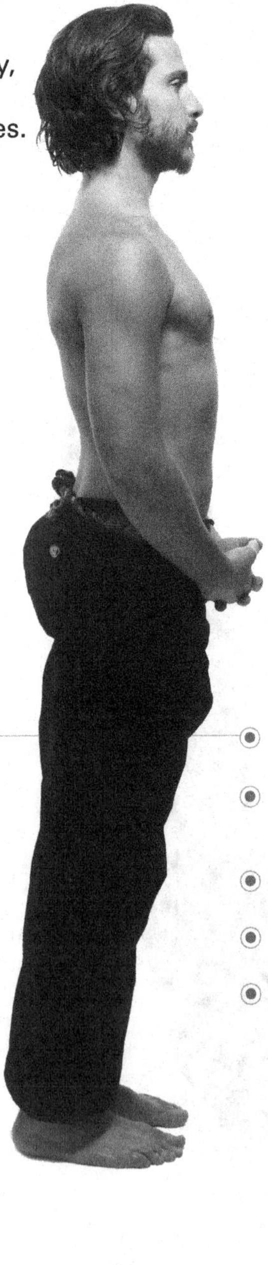

Fig. 5.10: Basic Stance

◉ Breathe normally.

◉ As you stand, align your body from feet to crown.

◉ Feel your energy flowing down to the ground.

◉ Push the sky with your head.

◉ Align your feet and bend your knees slightly.

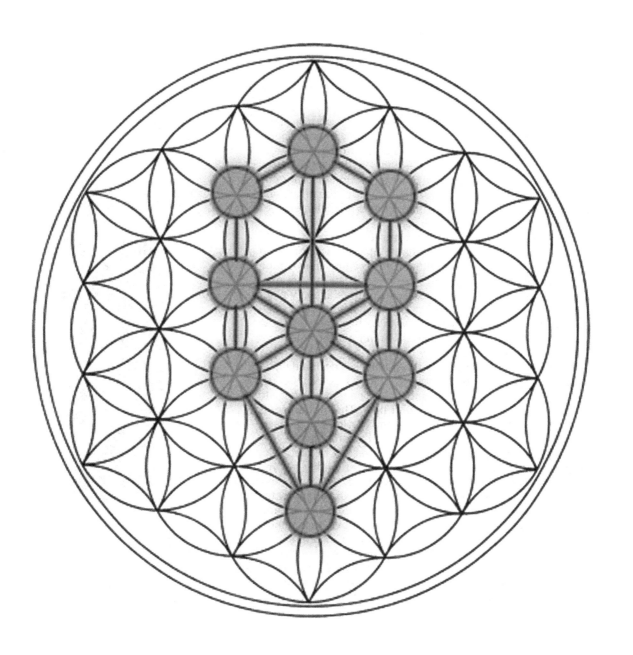

Chapter 6. *The Swimming Dragon*

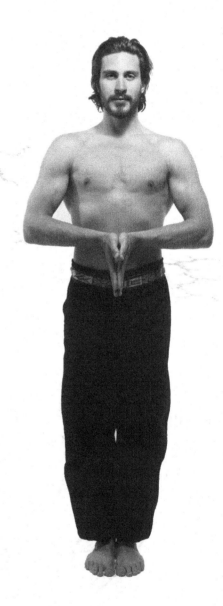

The Swimming Dragon, another chi kung adaptation, is especially beneficial for strengthening the legs and stimulating spinal vitality. It also helps to unlock the pelvis from the ribcage. In fact, it is a unification exercise—it works the entire body. Likewise, as a mythic creature, the Oriental dragon incorporates all elements in one. A dragon combines the fire (breath), metal (scales), and water (swimming), and utilizes the elements of heaven (it flies) and earth (it slithers).*

When I use this form, it delivers me to an alternate world and makes me think of Taoist shamans, Shaolin warriors, and legendary immortals. It is not difficult to imagine the bygone days of mystery, monastery, and martial arts. The muses may have been stripped from their caves by bulldozers and city planners, but the mythic wilderness is alive inside our skins. The dragon symbol has deep resonance with us because somehow we know we are more than just hairless orangutans. Life is more than just punch-clocks and grocery bills.

As mentioned in the Introduction, gravity is like a hand pushing down on our heads. The Swimming Dragon creates a powerful double helix—an ascending and a descending current—to help us shrug off the harmful effects of time. The motion cools the body's bioelectrical system and sets the whole being at ease. This dragon gives us rooted confidence and a serene brow.

During this, as well as all other exercises, try to keep your mind and body relaxed. Breathe slowly and smoothly, as you become more comfortable with the exercise, try one deep inhalation as the arms rise. And one deep exhalation as the hands lower. Keep in mind that as your hands cross the midline, they change positions—the shoulders always move opposite the hips—and your whole body (except for your head) should always face forward. Your head should follow your hands.

This form, though broken down here into fifteen steps, is not long. It is done in one smooth movement over the course of two, slow and gentle breaths. Try to do three or four Swimming Dragons on each side, six to eight total.

---

*The five elements according to classic Chinese medicine are Wood, Fire, Metal, Water and Earth.

THE SWIMMING DRAGON IN FIFTEEN STEPS

1. Step One: The Basic Stance

Take your Basic Stance, then move feet and knees together. Your hands should be touching in front of the groin. Then slowly bring them up to prayer position.

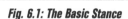

Fig. 6.1: The Basic Stance

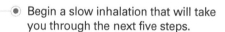

- Begin a slow inhalation that will take you through the next five steps.

- When the hands pass the heart, turn them upwards as in prayer.

- Keep your eyes forward and your brow relaxed.

2. Step Two: Hand Position

The following four steps are completed in one smooth movement: Bring your hands, still in a prayer position, up toward the right side of your face. The folded hands should pass by your head as if you are resting on a pillow and then continue smoothly to step 3.

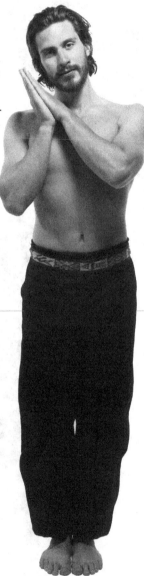

Fig. 6.2: Hand Position

- Keep your shoulders down, elbows wide.

- Keep your feet rooted.

- Imagine your spine as a serpent.

- When your hands pass the chest, begin your motion toward the chin.

3. Step Three: Reaching Hands Up

Slowly raise your hands past the right side of your head and extend, with your fingers pointing up.

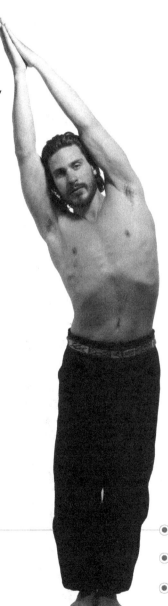

Fig. 6.3: Reaching Hands Up

- Continue the inhalation.

- Bring your arms all the way up.

- Imagine your spine as a serpent.

4. Step Four: Arms Over the Head

As your arms extend, move them directly overhead with your elbows straight.

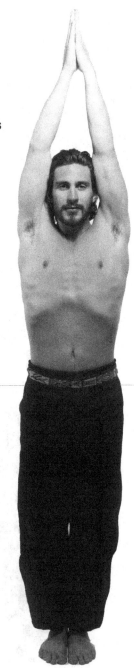

Fig. 6.4: Arms Over the Head

- Reach your arms high and bring them directly over your head.

- Keep your ribcage anchored.

- Try to lengthen the core muscles.

- Keep your feet balanced and centered.

5. Step Five: Arms Overhead Left

Trace your hands with your eyes as
they continue moving from the right
side to the left.

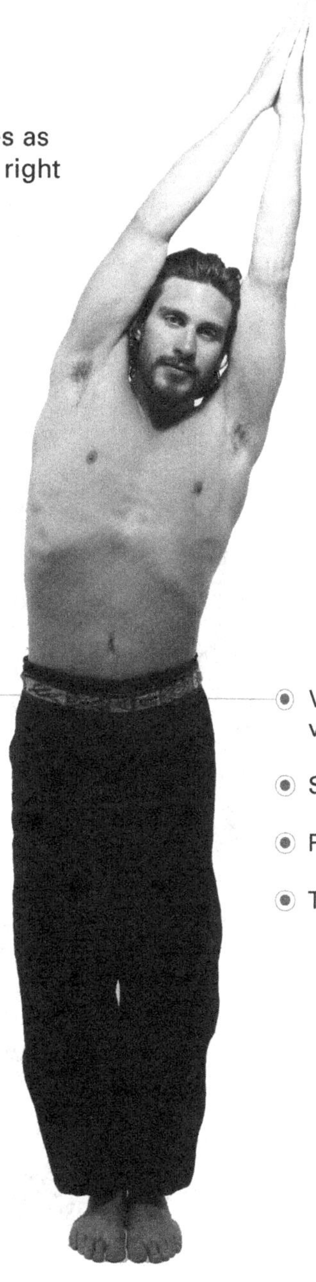

Fig. 6.5: Arms Overhead Left

- Visualize the space between each
  vertebra.

- Straighten out the knees.

- Feel the ribs unstick from the pelvis.

- Trace an arc across the sky.

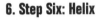

6. Step Six: Helix

Begin to exhale as you bring your hands down, point them to the right. Keep the palms together and flat. At this point, your shoulders should be opposite your hips. Exhalation will coincide with steps 6–9, completed in one smooth motion.

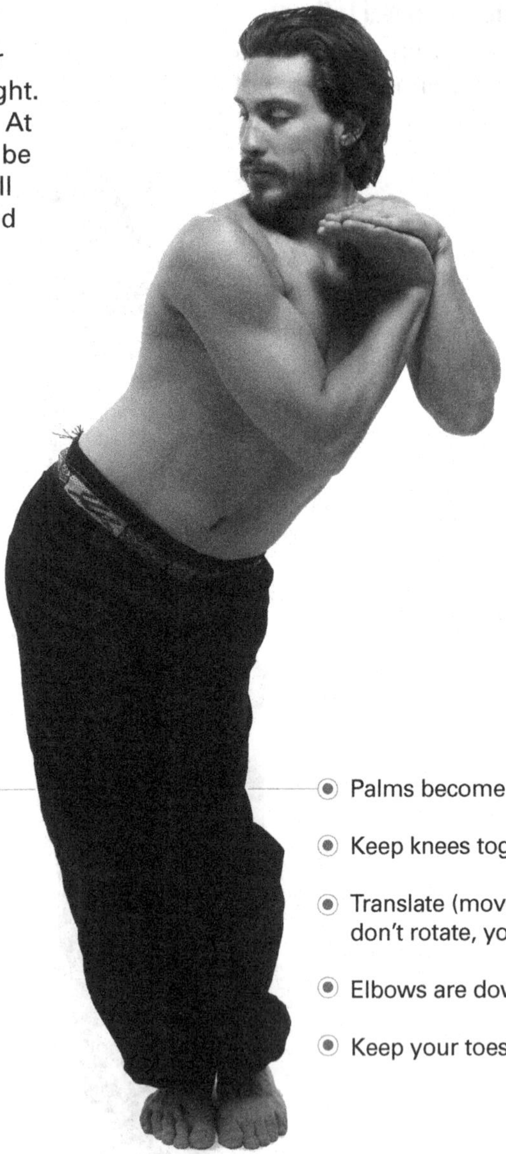

Fig. 6.6: Helix

● Palms become horizontal.

● Keep knees together.

● Translate (move laterally), don't rotate, your ribcage.

● Elbows are down.

● Keep your toes planted.

7. Step Seven: Dragon Flows Down

As your hands pass the head, begin to slide the shoulders to the right and the hips to the left, without twisting or rotating them.

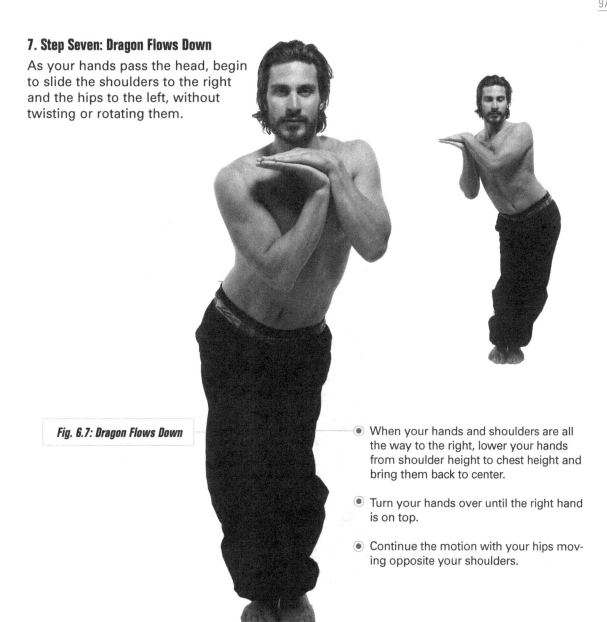

Fig. 6.7: Dragon Flows Down

- When your hands and shoulders are all the way to the right, lower your hands from shoulder height to chest height and bring them back to center.

- Turn your hands over until the right hand is on top.

- Continue the motion with your hips moving opposite your shoulders.

8. Step Eight: Dragon Snakes Left

When the hands reach the solar plexus, begin to trace them back to the left. Once again, as they cross the midline, the chest follows. When the hands have made it all the way, the chest will be to the left and the hips to the right.

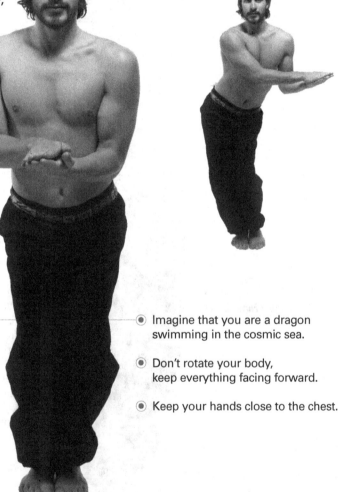

Fig. 6.8: Dragon Snakes Left

◉ Imagine that you are a dragon swimming in the cosmic sea.

◉ Don't rotate your body, keep everything facing forward.

◉ Keep your hands close to the chest.

9. Step Nine: Skiing Dragon

Lower your hands to the groin level
and cross the midline once again.

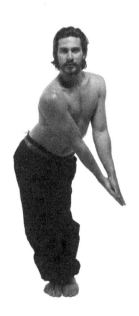

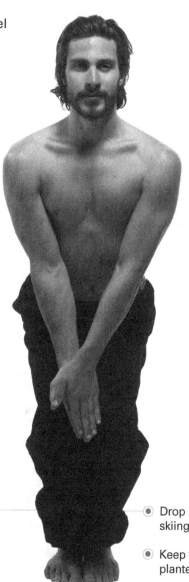

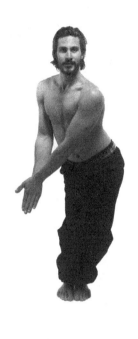

Fig. 6.9: Skiing Dragon

- Drop low into the knees like you are skiing.

- Keep your ankles relaxed and feet planted.

- Keep your whole body relaxed.

10. Step Ten: Second Breath, Second Pass

When your hands are on your right side, begin your second, deep inhale, bringing your hands up to the level of your chest.

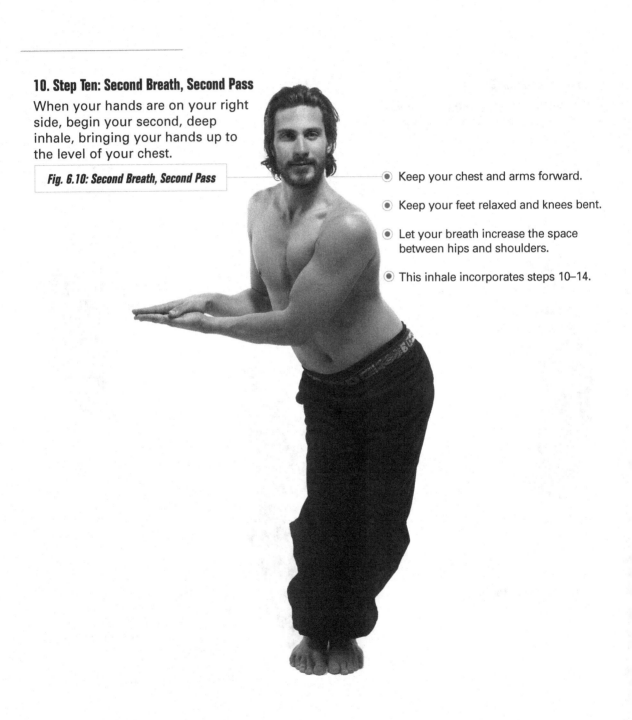

Fig. 6.10: Second Breath, Second Pass

- Keep your chest and arms forward.

- Keep your feet relaxed and knees bent.

- Let your breath increase the space between hips and shoulders.

- This inhale incorporates steps 10–14.

11. Step Eleven: Doubling Back

Cross your body again, hands and chest moving left and hips moving right.

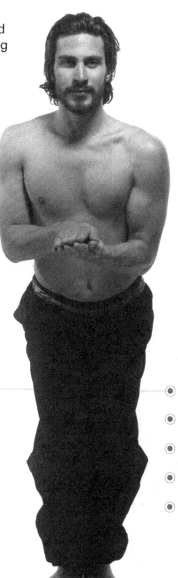

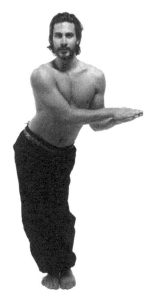

Fig. 6.11: Doubling Back

- Keep your hands close to your body.
- Shoulders down.
- Don't lean forward.
- Lift up from the chest.
- Visualize the double helix.

12. Step Twelve: Heading Home

Bring your hands up to the level of
your chin and then cross the body
again. The hands and chest move
right, and the hips move left.

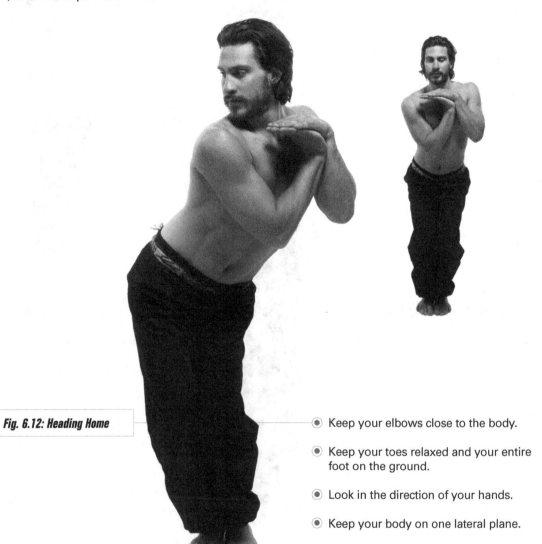

Fig. 6.12: Heading Home

⦿ Keep your elbows close to the body.

⦿ Keep your toes relaxed and your entire
   foot on the ground.

⦿ Look in the direction of your hands.

⦿ Keep your body on one lateral plane.

13. Step Thirteen: Giving Thanks

Continue to move your hands under your chin until they have reached the opposite side, to your right as in step 2. Begin to raise your hands up to the sky by passing them next to your face (like resting on a pillow).

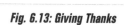

Fig. 6.13: Giving Thanks

- Put as much movement as possible into the spine and ribcage.

- Keep the palms of your hands together.

- Keep your elbows down as you cross your body.

- Keep your shoulders facing forward.

14. Step Fourteen: Giving Praise

Reach your hands as high as possible and lift up on your toes. Stretch to the sky, contract the butt, and make sure your feet are balanced.

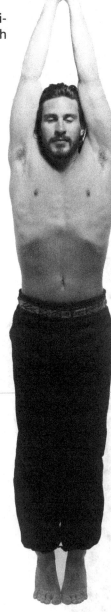

Fig. 6.14: Giving Praise

◉ Stretch as tall as possible.

◉ Make sure to keep your feet symmetrical.

◉ Keep your eyes forward.

15. Step Fifteen: Resting Dragon

Exhale. Slowly lower your heels as you open your arms to the side. Rest your body and take a few deep breaths to allow the energy to settle inside. Then repeat the exercise. When you are finished with one side, breathe a few times, and then gather the energy in your center, before practicing in the other direction.

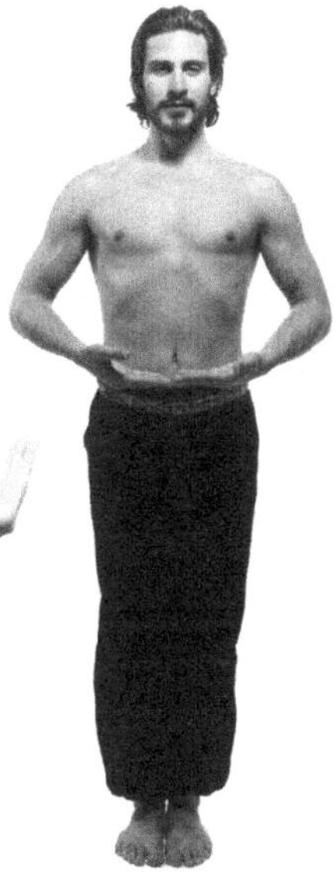

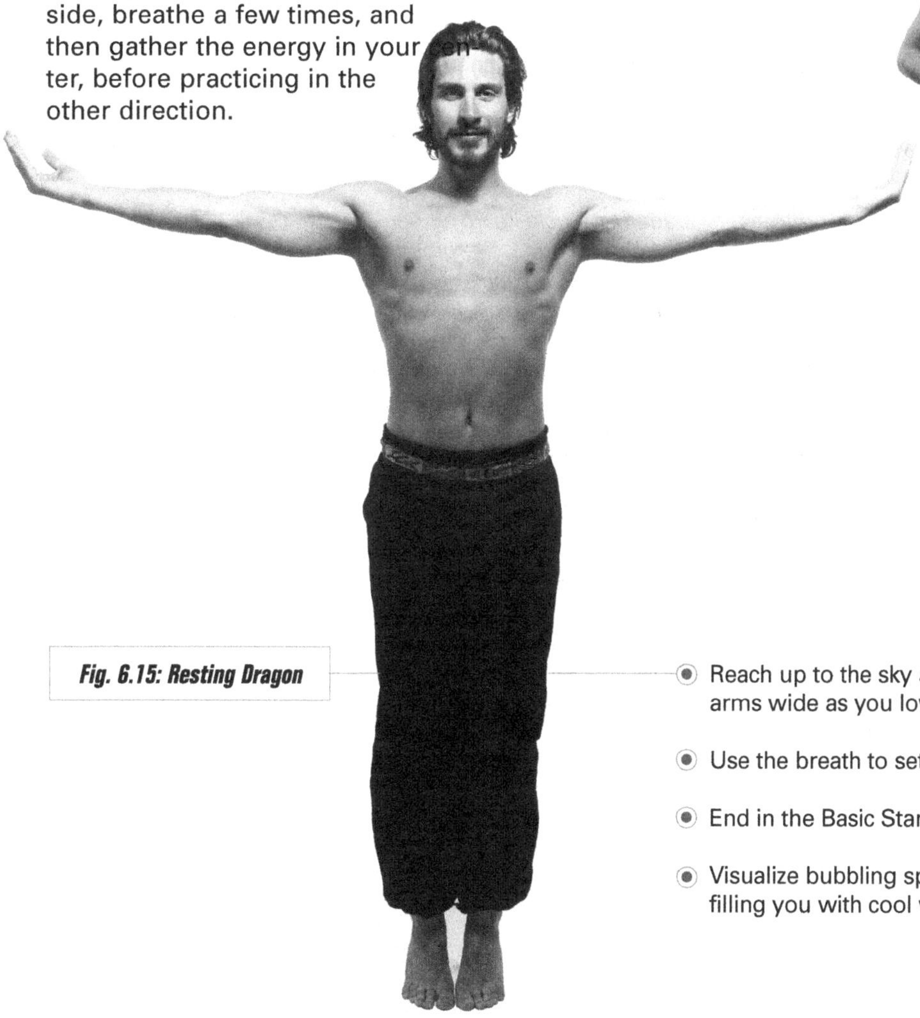

Fig. 6.15: Resting Dragon

- Reach up to the sky and then open your arms wide as you lower them down.

- Use the breath to settle the chi.

- End in the Basic Stance.

- Visualize bubbling springs in your feet filling you with cool water.

I AM A DRAGON, HOW DOES A DRAGON DO THINGS?

Depending on which country and century, dragon symbolism varies. The lore tells us two kinds of dragons exist—it is important to make the distinction.

The Western dragon is a gold-hoarding perversion of the id. A grotesque, overgrown, greedy child, the ego-terror personified.

In the East, the dragon is an infinitely wise, immortal creature. When you practice, get into the mythology of serpents and dragons. Imagine that you really are swimming in the cosmic sea, a place of infinite bliss and energy. Then confront yourself, "I am a dragon; how does a dragon live?"

Bring the dragon energy into your life. See how it feels to interact with the world not as a man or woman, but as a royal, immortal creature. Not in body, clothes, or accessories, but as spine, mind, and being. As you swim, slough off the skins that keep you bound to this world of illusion. Find the luminous and indestructible spine.

PART III

THE THERAPEUTIC SET:
EXERCISES FOR HEALING

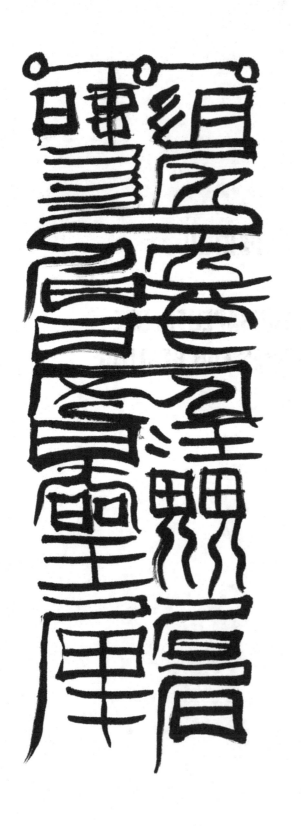

Remember, optimal health is not just about being strong and flexible, but also about being finely tuned and balanced. This is the true meaning of the Circle of Ease. Long-term practice leads to enhanced awareness of how to distribute healing energy, keep the spine free of distortions, and maintain balance within the viscera, bones, hormones, and skin.

At the end of the day, the most important thing is to feel good. As you start training and especially as you move on to the Advancement Set, you must give your body ample time to rest. The more you practice yoga and take care of your body, the more you will be able to control and subsequently heal almost all of your muscles. The aches, pains, and injuries become things of the past. You no longer abuse your body—you use it with grace and efficiency. And when something goes wrong, you can fix it.

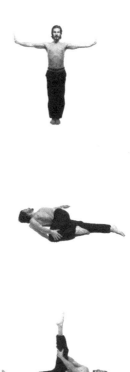

Opposite page: Talisman to cure all diseases. From Taoist Cannon. Author's calligraphy.

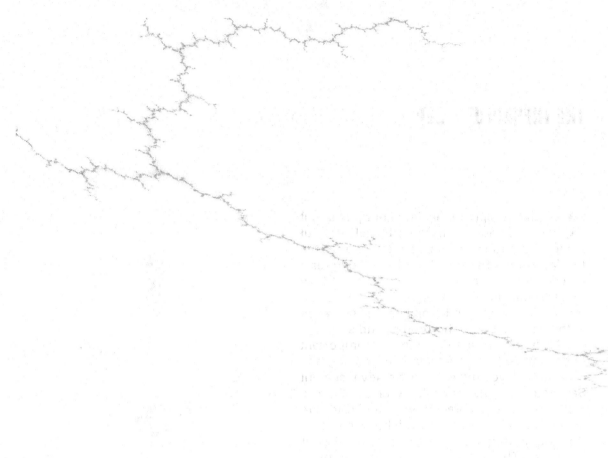

Let's face it, ours can be a traumatic existence. We are constantly bombarded with toxins, chemicals, and antibiotics in our food; we bear the stresses of driving, sitting at a desk, and walking on pavement. Most of us lack any kind of troubleshooting manual; we live our days almost numb to the attendant aches and pains, dulling them with aspirin or resigning ourselves to them as a part of life. Time goes by, and maybe we wake up one day and can barely move. The body, after years of neglect, finally quits, and then we are left asking, "How did I get this way?"

Let this be your troubleshooter.

Most common discomforts originate from one of six factors. Lack of breathing has already been covered in previous chapters, so let's address the other five:

(1) **Stress:** It's inevitable that life happens, and until we are aware of our bodies, we unconsciously take on external pain. We must learn to circumvent and interrupt the effects of stress. You can't end stress, but you can minimize its impact on you.

(2) **Overuse or Misuse:** Is your gym routine really helping you feel great, or is it just resulting in overdeveloped muscles? Have you noticed how you are sitting at your desk? How do you stand when you cook? Many common health problems have to do with the effects of routine activities that we do not pay attention to, or from using our bodies without intention, awareness, or mindfulness.

(3) **Objective Limitation:** Were you born with scoliosis or another medical condition? Have you ever had back surgery, knee surgery, or a broken neck? These are hard facts to deal with,

and you'll have to adjust your expectations of what you can accomplish accordingly.

(4) **Lack of Exercise:** Use it or lose it. In the old days, life was difficult enough to keep us fit. But now, unless we are working hard labor or consciously being active, we can't expect to stay in shape in the normal course of things. We will need to tune our bodies on purpose.

(5) **Obesity:** Excessive weight puts wear and tear on joints, limits locomotion, and stresses the heart. It also taps the organs and makes it hard to breathe.

Surprisingly, much can be done to alleviate all of the above. You can lose weight, bring awareness to movement, exercise, and feel better. As for objective limitations (preexisting conditions), it is just true that you probably won't re-grow a vertebra or replace the cartilage in your knee—unless you're an ultimate guru or a lizard.

Nonetheless, the good news is that there is almost always a margin for real improvement. For example, the first trick to overcoming objective limitations is to recognize the thought patterns that help to maintain the memory of the injury. Changing the phrase, "I have a knee injury" to "I *had* a knee injury" can make a significant difference in your mind and body. Then you must identify and focus on what can change, instead of constantly reaffirming the injury.

Step 1 involves creating positive thought patterns. Step 2 involves taking a realistic assessment of how much improvement is possible. Maybe that knee is never going to be 100 percent functional again, but from lack of exercise, lack of mindfulness, and negative thought patterns, its functional reality is only 20 percent, when its anatomical potential—the best that can be expected given the physics of the joint—is closer to 70 percent. That leaves a huge margin for real improvement. Step 3 is about applying your awareness, and Step 4 is practicing integrated exercise.

Achieving and maintaining real health is about prevention; so if any of these are true for you, and you have a chronic condition, it is paramount to stop the cause and change what needs to be changed at the source. Worry about treating the symptoms *after* that. There are some very tangible approaches available to relieving tension from the body. The old convention that symptoms are uncontrollable is actually false, because we have more capacity to heal and align our bodies than we ever imagined. You have already learned the Maintenance Set, which includes exercises to create and maintain a state of ease. Now let's consider how to heal the body from injury and illness.

TURNING ON, TURNING OFF

So much of life is based on action. When we exercise, we typically think about building stronger muscles. But the flipside of the coin is turning muscles off. The body works most efficiently when there is a balance between active and passive muscle groups. Think of it like a chord structure on a guitar. If some strings are sharp and others are flat and you strum them all, it will sound like discord and dissonance. Likewise, when the right balance between tension and relaxation is not achieved, we degrade our joints and stress our body. When all the strings are in tune, and only the correct ones are played, the instrument resonates with beautiful harmony.

While you should spend several days a week training, you should also spend some time each week practicing healing and restorative movements only. When you understand the language of the body, you can prevent a lot of basic problems at the onset. But no matter what you do, postures of rest and rejuvenation are absolutely essential. They restore the body to the point of balance. We may not be able to change the occurrence of occasional discomfort, but through therapeutic attention, we can keep things running smoothly. This begins when we learn to shut down, to be quiet, and do nothing.

SACRED SPACE

It is said that every cell in the body is regenerated within seven years. What is it then that keeps us bound to continue body disturbance patterns? Could it be that the thought-molecular matrix perpetuates certain unsubstantiated realities? If so, how can we hope to disrupt this cycle? How do we break the patterns? In other words, is quantum healing possible?

In order for healing to take place, we must create a sacred space—emptiness, both inside and outside. Depending on what you need, you can begin by taking a break from work. You can consult your doctor and begin to research different types of fasting. You want to give the body a break from its normal tasks so it can focus on healing. Some people fast with what is called a mono-diet, which could be as simple as just eating boiled rice. Other possibilities include the juice fast, raw foods, or maple syrup and lemon juice mixed with water. There is a wealth of information available on the Internet.

Once you have prepared your body with a fast, you will want to go through everything that you own. On a mundane level, this involves quite literally going through your closets and giving away or throwing out everything you don't need. You need to remove the chaos. Mentally and spiritually engage on a sort of vision quest in order to get back to those essential questions: Who am I? What is my highest purpose? What do I really want? What does the Universe really want with me? Spiritual and physical space will create the room for a breakthrough—balance in work, love, and health.

Next, seek some outside help. When we need new brakes or tires, we don't hesitate to drop the car off at the garage. Doesn't your body deserve the same? Assuming there are no urgent concerns that require medical attention, set aside some money and find an acupuncturist, an osteopath, a good chiropractor, or a deep-tissue massage therapist. Commit to seeing them for at least six weeks to work on everything you have neglected. In reality, it may take three to six months to really begin to transform.

Once you have removed the obstructions, you can start to heal. If you don't want to attach yourself to a guru or a specific spiritual path, you can develop your own mantras and healing meditations, focusing on what is most efficient and effective. There is a space—one of quiet, unassuming joy—where all disease vanishes as if the mere thought of it cannot exist within the presence of eternal being. You must go there as often as possible and stay there as long as possible.

1. RESTORATIVE POSES
General Relaxation
In the beginning, it is simple. There are three goals in the program: First, learn to sit and breathe; second, learn to rest on your back and let go of everything; and third, learn to walk like you're weightless.

When I first started my practice, it was nearly impossible for me to meditate. My muscles, back, and mind were so restless that the idea of sitting still for any period of time was unthinkable. Indeed, this is one of the reasons these exercises are so important. They prepare you for life. In fact, hatha yoga is the branch of yoga that was developed to prepare the human being for higher states of consciousness through physical exercise. In much the way that you need good suspension and tires on a jeep in order to go off-road, you need a good strong, lean, flexible body to enter higher states of consciousness.

One of the most important and powerful things we can do for our living system is learn to sit. There is an old Sufi proverb that sums it up: The student asks of the master, "Where did you learn such poise and awareness?" The teacher doesn't move from where he is sitting, but replies, "From a cat waiting outside a mouse hole."

Use the exercises to lengthen and free your spine and to unlock your movement potential. Then, even if just for ten breaths a day, practice the humble act of sitting. If after a few weeks or a few months, you find yourself able to be still—with your spine lifted and your head clear—you will have made a great stride in your overall health.

1.1. Sitting Meditation (comfortable position)

Wear loose, comfortable clothing and take off your shoes. Find a soft place, such as a blanket or yoga mat, and place a firm cushion under your buttocks. Fold one leg in, just under the groin and the other just outside of it. Let your hands rest where they will, and begin to practice D-breath. Then begin long and slow breathing and focus on emptiness. Float on the space between breaths. Use this awareness to tune into the heart, the pulse, and the viscera. Again, make sure you are breathing all the way out each time. Focus on the third eye and breathe into the spine, allowing it to elongate.

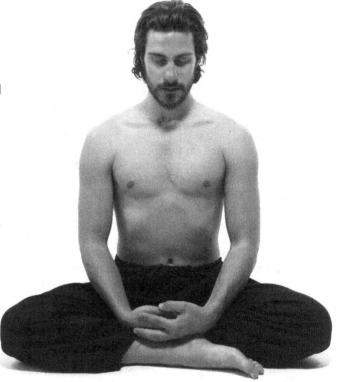

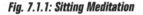

Fig. 7.1.1: Sitting Meditation

- Try to root the body, and lift up through all seven chakras.

- Lift the pelvis.

- Imagine the space between each of the vertebra expanding.

- To be more comfortable, slightly rock back and forth for a short time.

- You can visualize a candle flame or a circle or a mandala in your third eye (the sixth chakra between your eyebrows).

1.2. Walking Meditation

All this training is about awareness. But the idea is to
take this awareness from private, personal practice into
everyday life—life *is* the ultimate practice. Walking meditation is just what it sounds like: movement with mindfulness. Instead of scraping or heavily clunking the feet,
try to walk softly. To practice this, take off your shoes
and find somewhere flat, then lift one leg and bring it
forward. Touch the toes down gently, like you are a cat
or like you are walking on ice. After you have "tested the
ground," you can commit some weight onto that foot.
Try to develop a smooth transfer of weight from heel to
toe to heel to toe. Then repeat the process and walk
across the room. Work toward walking without having
any impact on the ground or your body.

Don't allow the head to fall
forward of the midline.

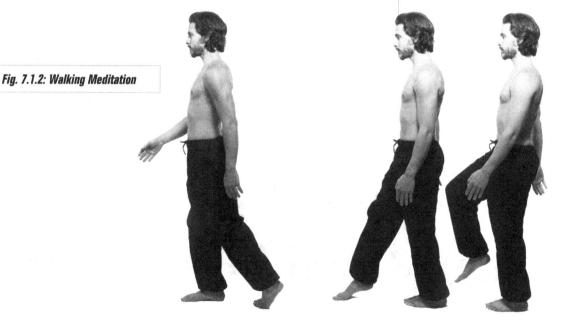

Fig. 7.1.2: Walking Meditation

1.3. Dead Body

Perhaps the most important of all these postures is the Dead Body or corpse pose. This is where you lie flat on your back and try to align—and yet relax—your whole body. Go through a mental checklist: shoulders, arms, hands, chest, abdomen, pelvis, legs, feet, brow, neck, head, and eyes. Imagine that every part of you is just sinking into the ground. Then you can visualize using your third eye. Just breathe naturally and let go of everything. You aim for a relaxed, supple, and responsive body. Take away any holding patterns, work through body-mind's memory, and just unwind. Return to the cosmic womb. Imagine you are a sponge soaking up the energy, wisdom, and vitality of the Universe. Rest and feel yourself fill with chi.

Fig. 7.1.3: Dead Body

- ◉ Relax everything and let your body sink into the floor.

- ◉ Rotate your shoulders back and relax the neck.

- ◉ If you want, you can massage your eyes, forehead, and neck.

- ◉ You may listen to the ambient sounds, but allow them to carry you away.

- ◉ Go beyond movement; meditate on the silent mover. The stillness beyond all form.

- ◉ Breathe.

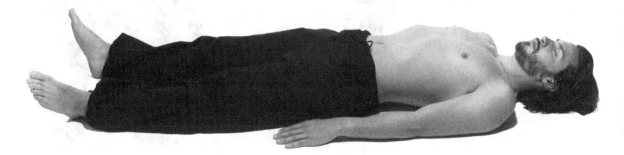

1.4. The Plough

After resting on your back, you can kick your legs over your head. Rock side to side and clasp your hands behind your back. Find the platform your shoulder blades provide and settle there to keep the weight off your neck. Inhale. On your exhale, stretch the muscles of the back of your legs gently to bring your knees down to your forehead. Inhale and hold. On your next exhale, slowly try to bring your knees down on either side of your ears. Breathe. Don't hold it in. After a while, you may even hear the energy moving. Now, straighten the legs out as much as is comfortable and reach your arms over your head; continue the stretch and breathe into it. Relax. Then slowly lower your legs back down. Don't flop, but maintain control, contact the floor with the spine, vertebra by vertebra, until your spine is flat. Keep the knees bent and then lower your feet to the ground. Slowly straighten the legs and return to Dead Body. Relax everything.

Fig. 7.1.4: The Plough

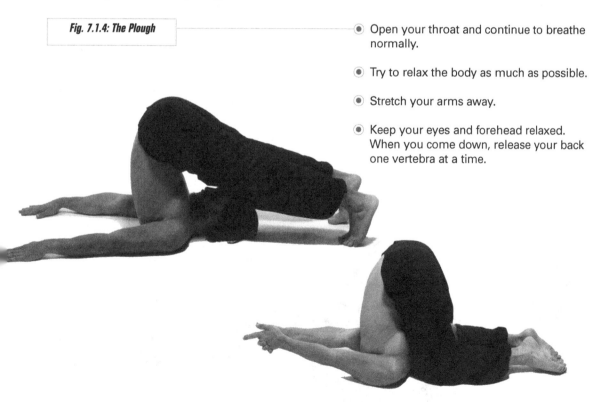

- Open your throat and continue to breathe normally.

- Try to relax the body as much as possible.

- Stretch your arms away.

- Keep your eyes and forehead relaxed. When you come down, release your back one vertebra at a time.

1.5. Spinal Twist

After a few minutes in the Dead Body, bend your right knee in and stretch it over your left leg to the floor, with the head and shoulders remaining flat. Breathe and stretch your hip and torso, unlocking your spine from the ribcage. You may hear your spine adjust. Reverse, stretching your left knee over to the right side. Breathe. Bend both knees into the chest and stretch your lower back. Lower first one leg and then the other to avoid stressing your back.

Fig. 7.1.5: Spinal Twist

- Relax your body and lengthen the spine as you twist to one side.

- Don't compress the lower back.

- Use the breath to help you stretch through the ribs.

- Adjust the stretch from your hip to your leg and up to your core.

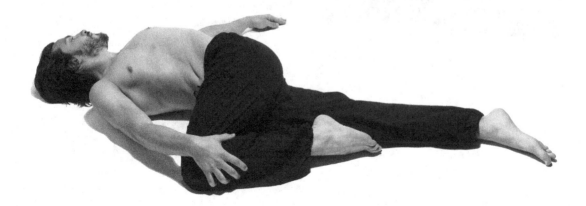

2. TROUBLESHOOTING

Now let's focus a bit on the specifics of how to fix common aches and pains. Aside from acute medical conditions, which may require the care of a physician, most chronic physical conditions are easy to diagnose and surprisingly easy to remedy. Just like a car needs an oil change and a tune-up after so many miles, our bodies need certain attention after a certain number of days. What follows are ways to give yourself a tune-up.

2.1. Pinched Nerve/Neck Spasm/Headaches

WHAT IT IS: You wake up to pouring rain, and adding to that, you slept on the pillow wrong. The sofa bed at your in-laws' is a killer ... Suddenly, it's intensely painful to turn your head to one side. This annoying occurrence is commonly referred to as a pinched nerve. Although it is possible a neuronal impingement is responsible, what is more likely is that you have an overly contracted neck muscle, typically the *levator scapularis*. This severe, involuntary contraction is referred to as a spasm.

WHAT TO DO ABOUT IT: Many common pains are involuntary contractions, which can set up what might be called a spasm or pain response. In short, it hurts; you tighten it, it hurts more, and you tighten more. What you want to do is relax the muscle. You can try taking the recommended dosage of an over-the-counter painkiller, such as aspirin or acetaminophen, or an anti-inflammatory like ibuprofen or naproxen. You can also take a hot shower or bath and put on comfortable clothing. You may want to do some self-massage or practice the neck stretches from the Basic Warm-Up. By slowly articulating the neck in all four directions (forward, backward, side, side) you may discover the root of the spasm—*if you can find it, you can unwind it*. After you have relaxed it as much as possible, lie flat on your back and lengthen your neck. Rest is essential for healing and allows all the energies of the body to flow.

Fig. 7.2.1 Fixing Neck Pain:

- Place a pillow or soft cushion under your knees.

- If necessary, bend the knees to release the lower back.

- Breathe fully and deeply, concentrating on a smooth and slow exhalation.

- Focus your awareness on sending healing energy radiating through the painful area.

- Practice slow, small movements—micro-movements—to see if you can gain information about the cause of the pain.

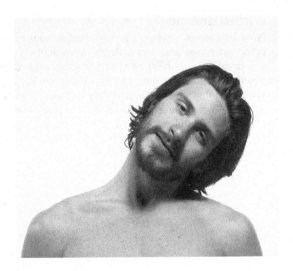

You can also swing your legs over your head and go into the plough (see fig. 7.1.4). Stretch your legs from side to side and try to locate the root of the spasm. This might be fairly painful, but remember, this is the release of the pain that lives in your body. If after a day or two it hasn't subsided, see your massage therapist or chiropractor.

2.2. Bad back, Lower Back Pain, Kyphosis (curvature of the spine)

As we have already discussed, ease of movement is achieved by a combination of tension and relaxation—the proper chord structure. Regular practice of the Basic Warm-Up and the Maintenance Set should relieve most of the nonobjective symptoms of back pain. Nonetheless, back problems occur frequently, and postural habits are hard to change. So let's take a closer look at what you can do about it.

2.2a. Lower Back Pain

WHAT IT IS: Lower back pain is often caused by a combination of weak abs, contracted core muscles, and tight or overdeveloped muscles in the buttocks, hip, and lower back. People often say "my back went out" when this is just a temporary inflammation of a permanent condition. Altering or fixing this problem often involves a combination of increasing flexibility, relaxation, and conditioning. Once again, finding a good massage therapist, chiropractor, or osteopath is invaluable.

WHAT TO DO ABOUT IT: Abs and Breath. It is imperative you practice the D-breath because it will allow you to bring the abdominals into shape. The back can be thought of as a foundation, and although it is designed to hold you up—the main muscles are called erectors—it should not work overtime. *Remember that muscles pull much better than they push.* When we lean on our back muscles, they are forced to act like a wedge or a splint. Eventually, the back just clicks in to autopilot, and then you have a bad spasm. However, the recruitment of the abdominals takes the pressure off the back and supports you from the front, and the breath lifts the spine and increases the space between each of the vertebra.

Flexibility. The abs and the lower back muscles should function like the front and back walls of a foundation, but there are also walls on the side, and in the case of the human body, the middle. These muscles are known as the *psoas* and *quadratus lumborum*. And both can be chronically tense or shortened. To relieve these muscles, you can practice the forward bend, the side stretch, and the spinal twists from the Eight Brocades, as well as the lunge positions in the Sun Salute. It is important to move the spine through all four directions, side, side, forward, and back. If you bring movement to an area, it will liven up. Think about it: algae grows in still water, not a running brook; stagnant parts of your body develop pain. Lower back pain may also be related to the depletion of kidney energy caused by lack of water, or even too much sex.*

---

*In Traditional Chinese Medicine (TCM), it is believed that the kidneys store jing or vital essence, which is finite and depleted by excessive sexual activity.

2.2b. Kyphosis

WHAT IT IS: Kyphosis is a medical term for a permanent curvature of the thoracic spine, which typically occurs in the form of what is commonly called a *hunchback* or *dowager's hump*. For most of us, it is not too severe or noticeable, but the fact is, as we age, gravity continues to push us forward of the midline. The greatest majority of our intelligence is focused forward, because this is where most of our outer anatomy is located. Few people ever think about arching back. When we do arch back, it is typically by hyper-extending one part of the spine, such as the cervical curve or the lumbar, but very rarely do we extend the middle of the back (the thoracic cavity), and this is precisely what must be done to relieve kyphosis.

WHAT YOU CAN DO ABOUT IT: The most important exercises to correct this kind of distortion are called back-extension exercises, and they are more fully described in the Advancement Set under Pilates-Style Exercises. One additional exercise, which can be done any time and almost anywhere, is the Desk Stretch.

The Desk Stretch. Find a stable surface approximately waist height (such as a chair or desk) and lean forward. Bend your knees, and place your feet about three feet away. Then place your hands on the surface. Tuck the abs, and with the shoulders extended, stretch down and attempt to flatten out the upper back. Focus the stretch on the thoracic region.

Fig. 7.2.2b: Desk Stretch

- Keep hands shoulder-width apart.

- Use the abs to stabilize your ribcage.

- Try to keep the lower back and neck neutral.

- Focus the stretch on the middle of the back.

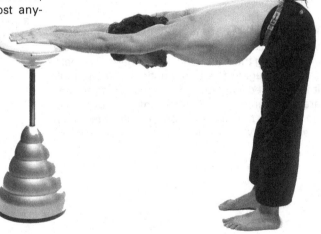

2.3. Sciatica/Tight Hips   Sciatica has become a catch phrase for a variety of conditions that can be caused by both a tight buttocks and hips.

WHAT IT IS: Sciatica is technically an impingement of the sciatic nerve by the *piriformis* muscle, which lies beneath the *gluteus maximus*. In the hip and buttocks, spasms and contractions can press on this nerve, causing extreme discomfort. It can cause pain down the back of the leg and throughout the hip and also in the lower back. Occasionally, herniated lumbar discs cause sciatica, but more often, it is simply tight muscles that lead to the pain.

WHAT YOU CAN DO ABOUT IT: Following the Maintenance Set and finding a good hands-on therapist is critical. You can also relieve sciatica by learning to place more weight in the quads when you stand. This way, the energy passes down to the ground and doesn't get stuck in the hips. This will also release lower back pain. There are also several good stretches that will help:

2.3a. Crossing the Leg

Most of us have one side of our back that is tighter than the other, and nine times out of ten, that is where "sciatica" flares up. One of the best ways to combat this is to cross the legs when you sit, with the ankle of your painful leg on the opposite knee. You likely cross your loose leg more often, so now cross the leg that is tighter—be sure to cross with the ankle over the knee. Crossing the legs one on top of the other can impinge the ligaments in the groin, whereas crossing this way—like making the number four—will stretch the sciatic region.

Fig. 7.2.3a: Crossed Leg Stretch

- Lift the lower back.

- Don't let the crossed leg move your spine; stay centered.

- Try to open from the hip.

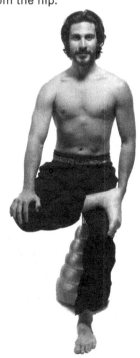

2.3b. Supine Sciatic Stretch

This same principle (external rotation) can be applied on the ground. Lie down face up and cross one leg over the other. Next reach around the other leg and clasp the hands. Curl up and press down on the opposite knee with the elbow.

- Use the abs to stabilize the stretch.

- Make sure that you cross the leg past the ankle.

- Lengthen the spine.

Fig. 7.2.3b: Supine Sciatic Stretch

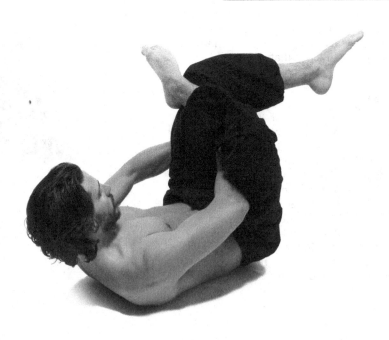

2.3c. The Sphinx

Another variation is called the Sphinx. Take a position on all fours, and then kick one leg up between the hands and turn it out so that the leg is resting on its lateral aspect. Slide the other leg back as if you are doing a lunge. Stretch.

- Try to keep the hips even.

- Lift up in the chest, but drop the hips.

- Don't strain the knee.

- Gradually feel it open in the hip.

2.3d. Self-Massage Finally, you can use a tennis ball to rub out the area. Lie on your back on a firm surface and place a tennis ball in your hip cuff. Roll side to side, up and down, and imagine that you are scraping the muscle off the bone. Trace the tension all the way around the hip cuff; when you find a tight area, breathe into it. Let your weight drop and the spasm release.

2.4. Feet

WHAT GOES WRONG: Neglect of our feet leads to a loss of range of motion, aches, pains, and the precursors to arthritis. For many people, the feet simply get us from place to place. We stuff them in shoes, walk where we need to, and don't give them much thought. As a result, many of the complicated muscles and bones in the toes and the ankles can become displaced or compressed.

WHAT YOU CAN DO ABOUT IT: Many of the exercises here work because of their simplicity. Articulating the joint with optimal awareness, redirecting the chi, and unsticking muscle groups are the keys to unlocking troubled areas. Remove your shoes and socks and practice the ankle stretches from the Basic Warm-Up. Recall the basic motions are to point, flex, and circle.

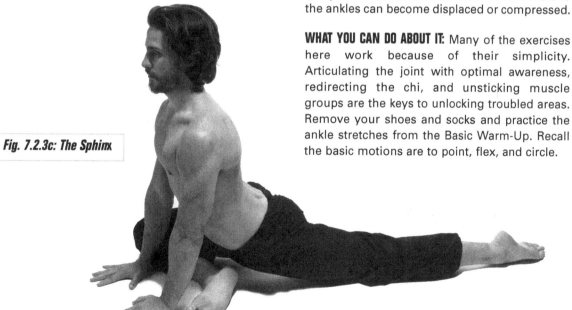

Fig. 7.2.3c: The Sphinx

2.4a-e. Ball and Toe

Here's a very simple but effective exercise. The intention is to unstick each moving part of the foot. You will try to move the toes independently (up and down) and also the body of the foot. By making each movement distinct, you will create patterns that are more efficient. Lie flat on your back and bend one knee into the chest. Straighten that leg up to the ceiling, point the foot, hold behind the knee, and begin to articulate the ankle.

Then, with the body of the foot in the same position, flex just the toes to the nose. Then flex the ball and the whole foot to the nose. Then point just the ball of the foot, but keep the toes extended. Return to toe flex, and then complete the process by pointing again.

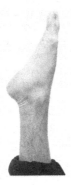

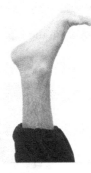

Fig. 7.2.4a: Point

Fig. 7.2.4b: Flex

◉ Try to point the whole foot and finish with the toes.

◉ Imagine there is a laser pointing through the whole leg and extending through the big toe.

◉ Keep the body of the foot on the midline.

◉ Imagine there is a hand holding the body of the foot so that just the toes can move.

◉ Focus on flexing all five toes equally.

◉ Extend out through the ball of the foot, even as the toes come up.

Fig. 7.2.4c: Ball

- Keep the toes up.

- Flex the foot in one small motion.

- Be aware of the midline.

- Don't crunch the ankle.

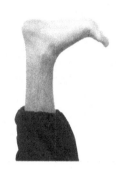

Fig. 7.2.4d: Toe Flex

- Use the motions to unstick the tendons in the foot.

- Imagine you are a cat stretching its paw in the window.

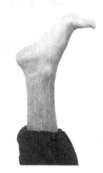

Fig. 7.2.4e: Toe Point

- Extend through the big toe like you are pointing a laser.

- Lengthen the whole leg.

- Straighten the knee and reach through the hip.

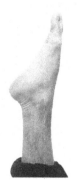

The Ball and the Toe and the Ball and the Toe

These foot exercises are best summarized by a rhythm. Starting with the whole foot pointed, flex just the toes so that the ball of the foot is pointing to the ceiling (ball), then flex the whole foot and toes up (toes), then point just the ball (ball), and finally point the whole foot (toes). Repeat ten times on each side and focus your awareness on the rest of the leg.

2.5. Carpal Tunnel Syndrome

WHAT IT IS: Carpal tunnel syndrome (CTS) is technically an impingement of the radial nerve by the *pectoralis minor muscle*. But like sciatica, it becomes a catchall term for various types of wrist and arm pain. The carpal tunnel is the area under a band of connective tissue that covers a bony groove (eight, tiny carpal bones) and forms the gateway of the wrist. When muscles are tight and wrist extension is not practiced, this highway can become bunched up, causing pain, tingling, and even numbness.

WHAT TO DO ABOUT IT: The treatment of CTS involves several factors. The first is to identify movement inefficiencies. Is there something that you are doing at the office, at work, or at play, that is routinely aggravating the area? If you must engage in this activity, can you prevent further aggravation of the problem by moving more consciously? At times, surgery is necessary, but only as a last resort.

The second thing to do is to find a good massage therapist and get some solid, deep-tissue work on the chest, biceps, forearms, and hands. After this, you should feel significantly better and ready to practice the following exercises:

2.5a. Wrist Extension

Repeat the wrist exercise from the Basic Warm-Up by using your opposite hand to stretch your lower arm with palm up. Try to stretch the hand through various angles.

Fig. 7.2.5a: Wrist Extension

- Take it slow and feel the various lines release.

- Feel the stretch from the wrist all the way to the elbow.

- To maximize your stretch, rotate the wrist in different directions.

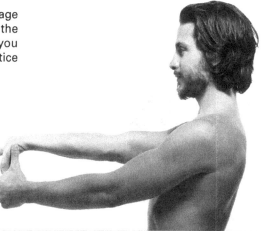

2.5b. The Cosmic Being

Take a comfortable stance and make sure to align your hips, shoulders, and head. Then open arms wide like a cross, palms down. Reach out as much as you can through your shoulders and elbows as you flex your hands and point your fingers to the sky. Don't let the shoulders break back; instead, breathe and reach out.

These postures of relaxation can become part of your nightly ritual. Before you go to sleep, it is likely you lock the doors and then turn off the light. Add to your nightly routine the means to rid your body of the day's tension, erase the stress, and restore the scales to zero. This way, not only will you sleep better, but you will also wake up with your body clear and free from the stress of yesterday.

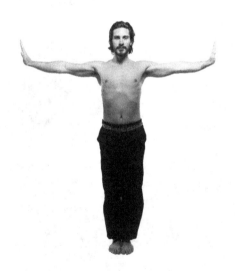

- ◉ Reach the arms as wide as possible, elbows pointing back, palms down.

- ◉ Flex the wrist and bring the fingers up, so they are pointing to the sky.

- ◉ Lengthen through the shoulder blades.

- ◉ Work through the tingling sensations.

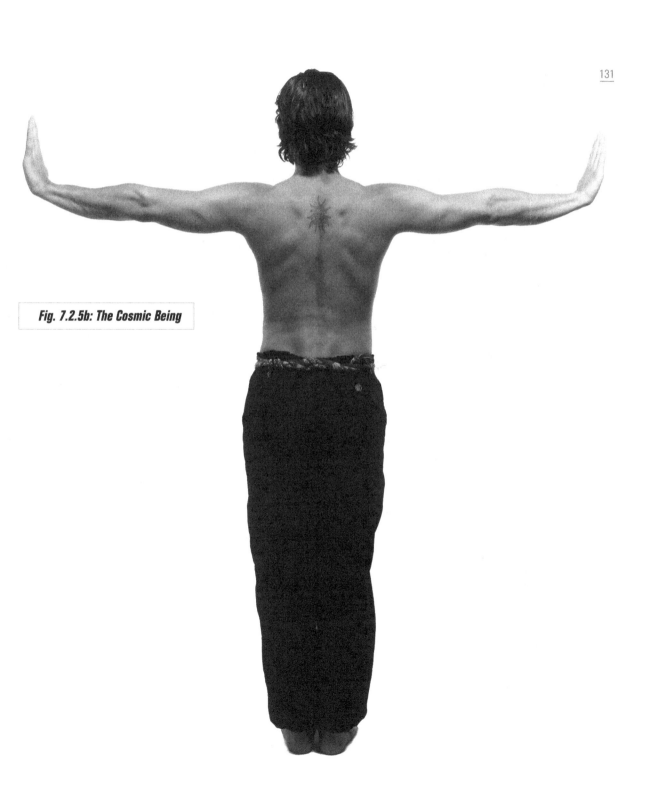

Fig. 7.2.5b: The Cosmic Being

Chapter 8. *Nutrition*

You can have the most high-performance motorcycle in the world, but if you put water in the gas tank, it won't run. Likewise, the body needs quality raw materials to sustain optimal function, to heal, and to allow for maximal efficiency. Diet is of profound importance and is critical for realizing a state of weightlessness. Without food, water, and oxygen, our bodies are incapable of sustaining life. If the chi is not nourished, it can't flow, build, or grow.

There are innumerable theories of nutrition and nutritional plans, and certainly some are more appropriate for one person than for another. But some basic nutritional elements are consistent across the board. Surely, we all agree that food contains the most energy in its natural state—when it is fresh and well prepared. Processed foods, stripped and sometimes refurbished with nutrients, can be destructive to the body.

There are some striking correlations between diet and disease. Indigenous cultures develop acne, bacterial infections, and tooth decay at alarming rates after the introduction of white flour, processed sugar, and preservatives. Recently, sugar and caffeine intake has been linked to Attention Deficit Disorder (ADD). The antibiotics added to industrial meats can kill off intestinal flora and increase our susceptibility to allergies, indigestion, and colds. In addition, highly processed proteins and supplements—though potent—can be difficult for the body to digest and put the organs under unnecessary stress or lead to indigestion and constipation.

Now more than ever, it is important to eat consciously and choose foods healthy for our bodies and the environment.

The guidelines set out in this chapter are based on personal experience and extensive research. They are designed to help you navigate the minefield of fad diets and toxic foods. Essentially, the dietary recommendations are based on a back-to-nature concept: we are the healthiest when we eat organic foods in their natural state.

- Eat organic, local, and seasonal.

- Try to limit processed foods.

- Eat sufficient greens.

- Don't eat too much.

- Make sure what goes in comes out (fiber).

- Stay away from preservatives.

- Stay away from sugar.

- Try to limit portion size.

- Drink plenty of water.

- Savor your food.

- Only eat when you are hungry.

VEGETARIAN DIETS

For some people, abstaining from meat is an ethical decision; for others, it is a political means of lobbying against a cruel industry; and for others, it is a health decision. If you are a vegetarian for health reasons, and it is the diet that makes you feel the best, then you are making the right decision. If you don't want to support big slaughterhouses, then you may want to consider local, grass-fed, and organic meats. As for the ethical concern, I hear you. I was a vegetarian for years and felt reasonably healthy. I figured that I was saving other living beings and leading a more compassionate life. There is truth to this, and it is noble, but don't allow your own health to suffer as a result. If you feel better, stronger, and healthier eating meat, then go ahead, but show sacred reverence for the animal sacrificing its life for yours.

Consider the fact that life lives on life. Imagine an old growth forest or jungle. What happens when a tree dies? Bacteria and fungi decompose the tree. New vegetation finds support and nourishment in the organic matter and then provides a source of food for other organisms like herbivores, which are eventually taken by predators. Ultimately, all die and are recycled back into the environment.

By only eating vegetarian foods, you may be limiting the complexity of life you take, but you are not removing yourself from the equation. Life lives on life. If you have struggled with this dilemma but feel healthier when you eat (organic) meat, it may help to consider that the energy of the animal—energy can neither be created nor destroyed—is being put to good use; it is being transformed.

After years of being a vegetarian, I ate a steak of black elk that a friend of mine shot with a bow. That night, I dreamed that I was that elk moving through the Northwest woods. The meat completely agreed with my body, and though the animal died, it filled me with inspiration, power, and energy. Following that experience, I started to consciously savor organic, and whenever possible, wild meat. And I have never felt healthier. The choice is up to you.

It is a great service to be a vegetarian, but it is not for everybody.

OMNIVOROUS SUSTAINABLE DIET

Vegetarians need to take special consideration to ensure they are getting enough and the right kinds of protein.

The following foods are listed in terms of super foods, acceptable foods, and those that should be used sparingly. If possible, eat exclusively from the super-foods list. But each person has a particular physical makeup, so it is important to look at the categories and choose the foods that resonate with you. It is important that you eat what you like and what is available in your region. Find your own personal building blocks for optimal health. For many of us, it may also help to do a round of probiotic supplements or cultures. These "good" bacteria can really help to restore the balance of intestinal flora and often alleviate symptoms such as allergies and indigestion.

SUPER FOODS

- All wild-caught, low-mercury fish
- Grass-fed organic meats (excluding pork)
- Free-range and organic chicken and eggs
- Goat cheese, goat milk
- All leafy greens (broccoli, kale, lettuce, swiss chard, collard greens, spinach, etc.)
- Whole grains (brown rice, millet, quinoa, barley),
- Beans, especially lentils, butter beans, and adzuki beans
- Olive oil, sesame oil, grape seed oil
- Maple syrup, honey, Agave nectar
- Spelt flour
- Seasonal fruit, especially berries
- Yerba mate tea, green tea, herbal tea
- Coconut water

ACCEPTABLE FOODS

- Whole wheat breads
- Pasta
- Tomatoes, eggplants, peppers
- Organic cow-milk cheeses, yoghurt
- Ice cream
- Organic sugar
- Organic butter
- Nonorganic oils
- Nonorganic vegetables
- Organic fruit pies
- Organic dark chocolate
- Organic dry red wine
- Organic espresso

USE SPARINGLY

- White flour
- White sugar
- Processed foods
- Processed oils
- Industrial meat, fish, and poultry
- Heavy, nonorganic desserts
- Pork
- Soda
- Alcohol

Note: Many foods have not been included on this list; please use your discretion.

It's possible to have different modes of being for different times in your life. Because each day, week, and season is different, it's important to eat what nature provides and also to be able to enjoy life's abundance—don't be too uptight. Think positively about your food and enjoy what the earth offers.

TYPES OF DIETS

For general purposes and for balance and enjoyment, diet can be broken down into these four modes:

1. Cleansing

2. Optimal Leanness

3. Sustainable Comfort

4. Bon Vivant *(holiday feast mode)*

For instance, in a given week, I may spend Monday cleansing, Tuesday and Wednesday in optimal leanness mode, Thursday and Friday in sustainable comfort, and Saturday and Sunday in bon vivant. When I get back to Monday, I have completed a cycle, but I have not gained or lost weight. Now depending on where you are with your weight-loss and optimization goals, you might need a different ratio.

Let's define each diet.

1. Cleansing

During a cleansing, you are eating very little food. Emphasis is on an elixir of organic lemon, maple syrup, and water with some cayenne pepper. You may also have fresh fruit juices, steamed vegetables, and small amounts of fish. Yerba mate as well as pep-permint and other herbal teas are acceptable, but other stimulants are avoided.

2. Optimal Leanness

During this period, food intake is kept to a minimum, perhaps a piece of fruit for breakfast, some salad, and a light dinner with fish, vegetables, and a small amount of healthy carbohydrates. I advise drinking a fair amount of herbal tea with honey in it or to make lemonade with maple syrup and organic lemon juice. You are eating about 90 percent of your full capacity, but all food comes from the super-food list; sugars, refined carbohydrates, and other sweets are completely avoided. This is your ideal diet for training, healing, and mental clarity.

3. Sustainable Comfort Mode

In this mode, you eat 100 percent of your output, so in theory you maintain your weight and leanness. Most foods come from the super-food list, but you may also mix in foods from the acceptable list— pasta, organic butter, and fruit pies. You can also have one sweet a day—*at most*—from the "use sparingly" column. In comfort mode, one to two cups of coffee a day is fine, as is an occasional glass of dry, red wine or high-quality distilled liquor.

4. Bon Vivant (feast mode)

Let's party! This mode should be indulged sparingly and enjoyed to the fullest. However, you should only treat yourself to it when your body is in excellent condition and the organ energies have been rejuvenated through a continuous period of optimal leanness. It is quite possible that after eating from the super-food list, your cravings for lesser foods will abate, and bon vivant mode will mean eating a big organic steak, a fat bowl of pasta, or whatever you crave. What's important is that you enjoy life and that you get healthy enough to tolerate some slightly less healthy foods. At festival time, put aside your guidelines and get loose. Food is one of the great joys of life for our species and our culture, so at the appropriate times, by all means enjoy— eat, drink, and be merry.

Getting in touch with your personal diet and what makes you feel the best is the key to eating well and living healthfully. Listen to your body and pay close attention to your digestion. If something causes you to be gassy, stuffy, constipated, or heavy, it probably doesn't agree with your personal chemistry. This is a direct feedback from your level of vitality. As you monitor your intake, you can form a list of your own super foods, and you will learn to vary your dietary choices to enjoy the bounty of life without compromising the feeling of weightlessness that you are cultivating. For optimal clarity, an optimal diet.

It also helps to have a positive attitude about food and, whenever possible, to prepare it yourself. Learn to get involved in the joy of cooking as well as the process of selecting the most high-quality foods. You may notice a little spike in your grocery bill, but it will most likely be accompanied by a long-term dip in your medical costs.

As you bring awareness to your body and your life, it will naturally extend to your food. If you have the taste for it, seek out wild foods, or get involved in gardening—whatever it is, the sooner whole, fresh food gets to your table, the better.

Becoming fully human is about being an artist of life, from the tiniest detail to a monumental act. Turn the TV off and bring conscious intention to your kitchen and dinner table. It is one of the greatest sensual and cultural joys in the world.

Optimal nutrition has less to do with moment-to-moment fads and diets and more to do with long-term healthy decisions. A moderate diet filled with whole foods, balanced intake and plenty of water should supply your with all the nutrition you need. It may be slightly more expensive, and take a little more time to prepare, but good food is the foundation of a healthy body. Breath and nourishment are the two building blocks of chi.

PART IV

THE ADVANCEMENT SET:
EXERCISES FOR MASTERY

WEIGHTLESSNESS

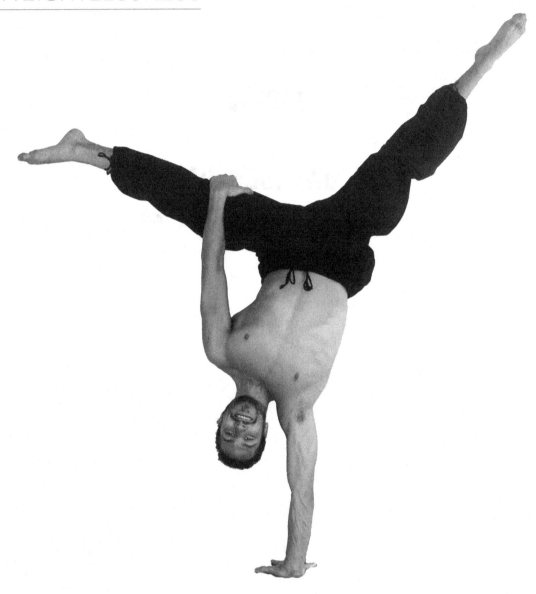

W e are training to stay centered in the circle of ease, the *weightless zone*. There is a legend in martial arts film lore about an ancient fighting style known as the Solar Sun Stance. This style would allow you to fight against any other method, because it was able to transcend yet include other more partial forms. Like this mythic training, the exercises in the Advancement Set are developed as a rigorous discipline that will lead to permanent, unbroken awareness. When you can bend, twist, and flip your body without losing your center, and maintain smooth breath and a clear mind, then nothing can touch you. You pass all trials and become like the ancient immortals: able to learn and do anything you wish with grace and efficiency.

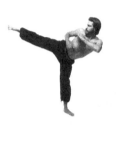

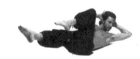

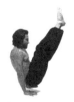

Chapter 9. *Hatha Yoga*

The word yoga comes from the Sanskrit root *yuj*, which translates to *yoke* or to *unify*. In practical terms, it is about unifying the subconscious and conscious aspects of the mind and gaining voluntary control over the body. Essentially, integration. In the metaphysical realm, yoga is the process of stripping away the delusions, physical restrictions, and behaviors that prevent us from identifying with universal energy rather than the limited self. In yogic cosmology, the goal is to overcome Maya (illusion) and realize Brahman (universal consciousness).

Modern yoga is largely derived from the work of Pattanjali, an ancient sage whose compiled *sutras* linked together and systemized what was already in existence. Scholars have a difficult time determining exactly when he lived, or if he was even one person. But along with the Bhagavad Gita, and the Vedas, the sutras are one of the key books in understanding the spiritual foundations as well as the physical practice of yoga.

Asanas, or postures, are just one part of this comprehensive discipline, which includes karma yoga (the yoga of action), raja yoga (the yoga of the mind), and bhakti yoga (the yoga of devotion). In the west, yoga usually refers mostly to hatha yoga, the branch that deals primarily with the postures.

Most beginners to yoga will notice that during practice there is a little voice in their head screaming, *Let me out of this pretzel!* As B. K. S. Iyengar once said, "For the first six years, I only practiced the asanas ... what can I know of philosophy, without health?"

Over time, these postures help lead us to self-knowledge, at the very least, by teaching balance, discipline, and patience. They likely evolved as tools to assist in meditation. As anyone who has ever sat still for more than fifteen minutes can attest, all kinds of aches and pains are common in the practice. Yoga postures help to prepare the body for sitting comfortably in meditation, a prerequisite for entering deeper states of consciousness. They are believed to prepare the body's so-called *psychic channels* to handle the higher wattage of advanced spiritual realization.

Yogic practice also helps bring into control our primal, instinctual urges; it sensitizes us to the effects of an impure life, giving real, sensory feedback to the things that prevent us from achieving health and the experience of weightlessness. This is because yogic observation allows us to become aware of internal organs, movement patterns, and how thoughts ripple through the body. The meditations, reflections, breathing exercises, chanting, and movements are intended to be a science of mind with the goal being presence, centeredness, full awakening.

The *Yoga Sutras of Pattanjali* describes yoga as "the intentional stopping of the unintentional chatter of the mind" and goes on to list what is commonly referred to as astanga (also ashtanga) yoga or the Eight Limbs.

THE EIGHT LIMBS*

- Yama (the five abstentions): nonviolence, nonlying, noncovetousness, nonsensuality, and nonpossessiveness.
- Niyama (the five observances): purity, contentment, austerity, study, and surrender to god.
- Asana: literally means seat and, in Patanjali's sutras, refers to the seated position used for meditation.
- Pranayama (suspending breath): *prāna*, breath, plus *āyāma*, to restrain or stop. Also interpreted as control of the life force.
- Pratyahara (abstraction): withdrawal of the senses from external objects.
- Dharana (concentration): fixing the attention on a single object.
- Dhyana (meditation): Intense contemplation of the nature of the object of meditation.
- Samādhi (liberation): merging consciousness with the object of meditation.

Though not necessarily religious in nature, traditional yoga practice always adheres to these moral and ethical constraints (yamas and nyamas). This is a strategy for calming the mind. Naturally, it will be hard to concentrate if we make a lot of enemies. If we are stealing for a living. Lusting all over town. Furthermore, these activities will ignite the fires of passion that takes us away from peace.

Of the yamas, the most important is usually considered to be ahimsa, or nonviolence. It can be argued that the others all flow from this fundamental abstention. Many practitioners believe that without the practice of the Eight Limbs and specifically yama and niyama, one is just doing acrobatics and is no different than a circus performer.

Another component of yoga is the understanding of the three *gunas* or qualities. These are: *rajas, tammas* and *sattvas*. Rajas refer to activity. Tammas to passivity. And sattvas to truth and clarity. Traditional yogis believe, and this is also at the foundation of ayurveda (the traditional alternative medicine of India), that the universe is made up of these three different types of energy. Yogis try to eat, work, practice, and act in accordance with sattvas—bringing stillness, truth, and clarity to their lives. Certainly, stillness and clarity are essential components of any focused practice.

So what is the goal of yoga? It depends. For some, it is just flexibility and greater body awareness. Through optimal attunement of the body, you transcend limitations, realizing that you are not a mere mortal form, but part of the immortal energy of the universe. Thus, we see beyond the illusion (maya) and enter the realm of pure being (Brahman). This is what is meant by union. The knower and the known become one. The practice of yoga allows us to expand our thoughts and see beyond the duality of life to the nondualistic, all encompassing cosmos, which in yogic terms is referred to as the Brahman. Or it might just mean getting a good, ego-bending workout.

ONWARD ASANA

The postures that follow are in the intermediate range, some slightly more difficult than others. Nevertheless, they are an important part of the language of the body. Studying these postures will prepare you for a variety of yoga styles. Please begin with a warm-up—your own sequence or any of those presented in this book.

---

*Definitions from Wikipedia, the Free Encyclopedia. http:www.wikipedia.org.

At the end of the chapter is a list of principles, guiding concepts for your practice. Mastering these principles will allow you to maximize the value of any class and will release limitless balance and flexibility from your body.

In all the postures, it is important that you breathe smoothly and control the eyes. Wandering eyes correlate with a wandering mind. Pick one spot on the wall and try to focus on that spot, only blink when you have to. It is recommended that you rest between the different groups of the postures. This means lie flat on your back and relax your entire body in a posture called corpse pose, or dead body. The period of rest should be no more than a few seconds or a few breaths, just long enough to unwind the body from a strenuous posture. At the end of the whole practice, you can spend about ten minutes in relaxation position. Then sit for a few minutes in meditation, observing the self, simply done by observing your breath.

ADVANCEMENT BREATHING

Pranayama or breath work is one of the eight branches of yoga, but for the purpose of this book, I will not get into these deeper practices. Of the various types of breathing, the most important for gaining flexibility, and for the general practitioner, is the natural, diaphragmatic breath, the D-breath... but with a few minor additions. It is not necessary to do breathing exercises that are more difficult until you've mastered normal breathing. This is like trying to do a handstand before you've learned to walk.

So what is the advancement breath? When you are deep in these postures, you will find that as you fill with air, your lungs expand (naturally), which makes the stretch more intense. The human tendency is to withdraw from this intensity and go forward again on the exhalation. This is analogous to going two steps forward and two steps back. Advancement breathing means that you maintain your awareness through the inhalation cycle, and then on exhalation, you actually go farther into the stretch.

Real progress in yoga only occurs with effort and mindfulness. You must be disciplined. In other words, don't allow yourself to be lazy. If you aren't trying, it doesn't count. Advancement breathing is one of the most effective means to regulate your mind and assure you are maintaining continuous presence. It makes you *show up*.

What follows is a comprehensive set of hatha yoga postures, which will prepare you to quickly integrate the asanas in Iyengar, Bikram, Shivananda, Dharma yoga—virtually any of the named schools.

Hatha yoga seeks to develop all parts of your being. Try to engage it with deep reverence. Apart from any religion, yoga practice should nonetheless be approached as a sort of prayer.

Before beginning, wear loose, comfortable, and minimal clothing, empty the bowels, and make sure it has been at least an hour since you have eaten. Begin with a ten-count practice, and then work up to fifteen and eventually twenty counts.

Always practice the exercises on both sides of your body. It is not so important that you follow the sequence, but if you want to work on a specific posture make sure you first complete a comprehensive warm-up. Advanced balancing poses can be dangerous for the hamstrings and back if your mind is not focused and your body not sufficiently prepared.

ON PRACTICE

I think that one of the most challenging and also rewarding things about yoga is that it reveals human potential. The more you practice, the more you will be able to realize the beauty and power of these postures. But there is no finish line. Every single day there is an opportunity to improve focus, anatomical integrity, awareness. To push the limit, while respecting the boundaries. I am and will always remain a student in the quest for mastery and liberation. Breakthrough, insight, inspiration, liberation—these are the rewards of a daily practice. It is okay to improvise, but be sure to balance things out. For example, if you do a back bend, be sure to counter it with a forward bend to decompress the vertebrae. Always work within your limits; there is no need to try a one-arm handstand before you can do a regular handstand, and don't forget to go slow and relax your mind. Breathing, imagining, and feeling are how you develop awareness. Take your time. Be present.

The Four Directions of the Spine

The following exercises are designed to maximize spinal flexibility. Always remember that lengthening through the joint attains the maximal effect of a stretch. Visualize the space between each of your vertebra expanding. When speaking of the four directions, it is worth mentioning a fifth direction, the center or axis mundi. Before proceeding, reach your arms over your head and stretch as high as possible—taller, up, up, up ...

- Clasp your hands together, but point your index fingers.

- Straighten the elbows as much as possible.

- Stretch one shoulder, then the other; then stretch both to the ears.

- Align the ribcage, keep the feet down, and imagine you are floating.

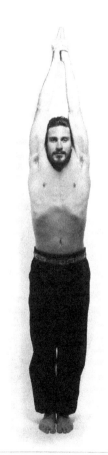

Fig. 9.1a: The Axis Mundi

STANDING POSES

Knees: to bend or not to bend? In the beginning, you will definitely want to bend your knees, as this will make standing/balancing postures safer and easier. As you progress, there will come a point where it will be important to work toward a straight, standing leg. To support a straight leg, you must contract the quadriceps (thigh muscles)—this protects your knees from hyperextension and improves balance and stability.

1. Side Bend

Stand with your feet together, knees straight, and your abdominals tucked in. Clasp your palms together and reach both arms over your head. Lengthen your shoulders as much as possible and reach up. Push your hip to one side and stretch over. Imagine that you are lengthening over a barrel.

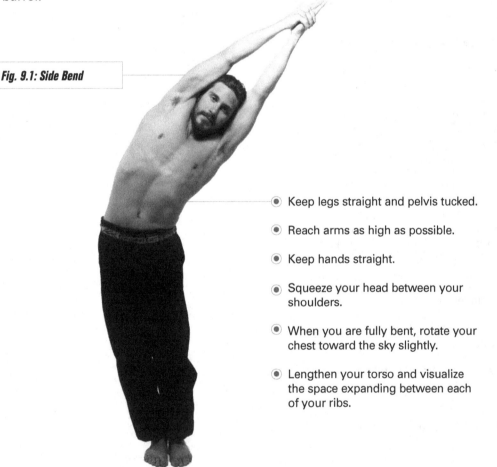

Fig. 9.1: Side Bend

- Keep legs straight and pelvis tucked.

- Reach arms as high as possible.

- Keep hands straight.

- Squeeze your head between your shoulders.

- When you are fully bent, rotate your chest toward the sky slightly.

- Lengthen your torso and visualize the space expanding between each of your ribs.

2. Back Bend

Return to center, reach your arms up, and squeeze your head between your shoulders once again. Squeeze your knees together and contract the abdominals to protect your lower back. Then arch your body and try to look behind you. Keeping your knees straight, feel the connection between your abs to your quads. Ideally, the stomach muscles should help hold us up from the front. Just as there are four walls in a foundation, the front of the body provides the front two walls and is necessary for stability. In this way, the body's muscles are using dynamic tension for support much like bridge cables and high-tech engineering do.

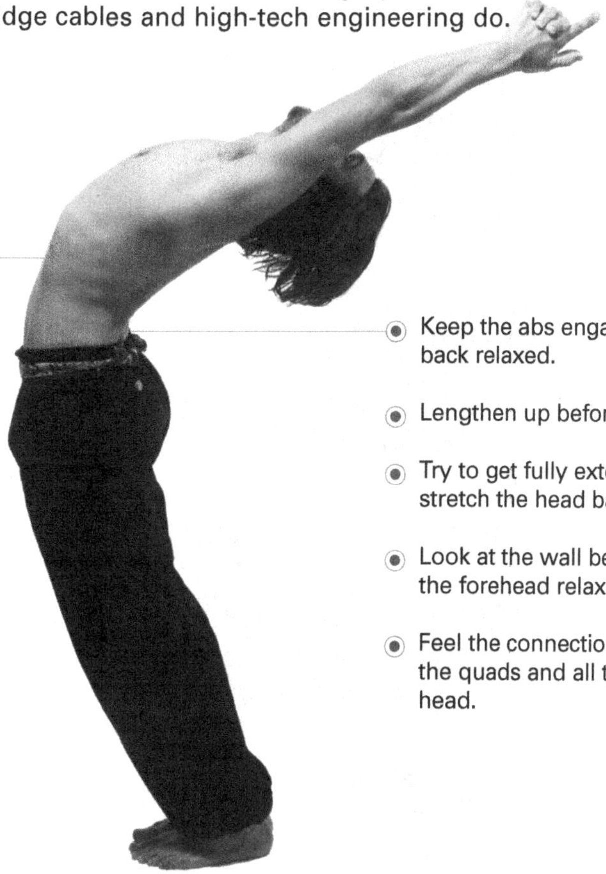

Fig. 9.2: Back Bend

- Keep the abs engaged and the lower back relaxed.
- Lengthen up before moving back.
- Try to get fully extended before you stretch the head back.
- Look at the wall behind you, but keep the forehead relaxed.
- Feel the connection from the abs to the quads and all the way to the head.

3. Forward Bend

Reach your arms over your head, palms facing out. Reach forward and keep your back straight as you fold down. Grab your heels and pull so that your chest goes against the thigh; lace your elbows behind your calf muscles, and allow your forehead to rest against your shin. If it helps, bend your knees a little but try to get a nice, long spine. Little by little, you can work on straightening your knees.

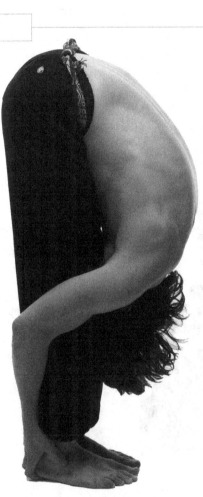

Fig. 9.3: Forward Bend

- Keep your abs engaged and lift your ribcage up and over your thighs.

- Lengthen from the lower back and feel the stretch from your sacroiliac joint through your whole spine.

- Continuously work on straightening your knees, but don't lock them back.

- Imagine that all the muscles in your legs are wrapping around your bones.

- Try to have equal weight on both feet.

4. Tree

Stand with your feet together on the mat. Straighten your left leg, tuck your belly, and lift your chest. Bring your right leg up the side of your left and rotate out so that you can place your foot heel-side-up against the inside top of your left leg. Adjust your heel so it is slightly more forward than the toe. Push forward with your pelvis and continue to lift the abs. As you balance, bring your hands into prayer position or lift your arms over your head.

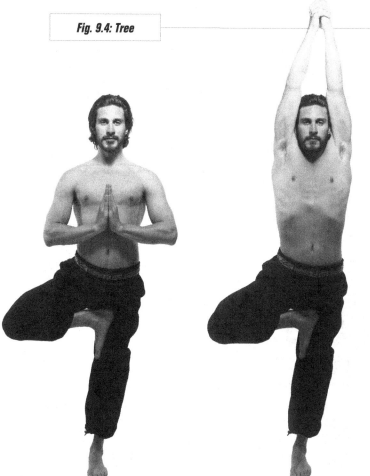

Fig. 9.4: Tree

- Always lift up and out from the spine.

- Contract the quads and push the floor with your standing leg.

- Continually push the bent leg back, but don't allow the pelvis to fall off-center.

- Keep your eyes forward and focused.

- Breathe.

5. Eagle

Bend down and cross your left arm over your right and interlace your
fingers. Bend your knees slightly and cross your right leg over the left.
Try to lace your right foot over your left calf. Sit down into the posture
as if you are sitting in a chair (don't go all the way to the floor).

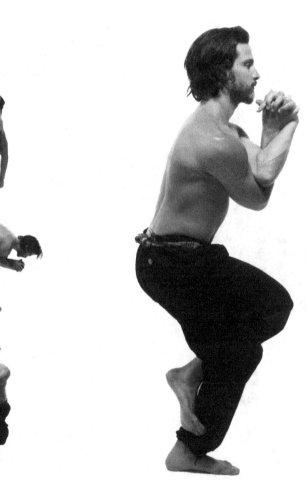

Fig. 9.5: Eagle

- ◉ Continuously push down through the hips and up through the chest.

- ◉ Lengthen the top of your head and tuck your chin.

- ◉ Don't allow your pelvis to fall off-center.

- ◉ Keep your chin tucked.

- ◉ Try to keep your whole body pointing forward.

- ◉ Bring your hands under your chin.

- ◉ Breathe.

6. Standing Bow

Return to center and straighten your left leg. Bring your right leg behind your body and grab the inside of your foot with your right hand. Keep the standing leg straight and reach straight ahead with the left arm as you hinge forward at the waist. Go down as far as possible but continue to push back with the leg that is up. Rest and complete the exercise on the other side.

Fig. 9.6: Standing Bow

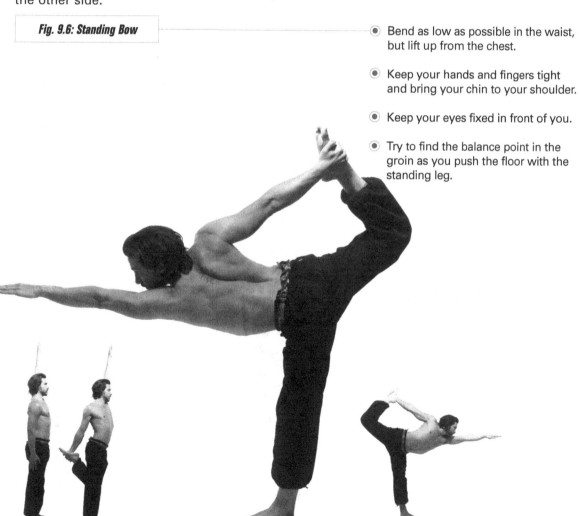

- Bend as low as possible in the waist, but lift up from the chest.

- Keep your hands and fingers tight and bring your chin to your shoulder.

- Keep your eyes fixed in front of you.

- Try to find the balance point in the groin as you push the floor with the standing leg.

7. Balance Stick

Return to center and reach both arms over your head. Straighten your
left leg and reach your right leg back slightly. Hinge forward at the waist
and balance. Try to get your hands and legs on one line, parallel with
the floor. Switch sides.

Fig. 9.7: Balance Stick

⊙ The key to this position is dynamic
tension. Point your foot and reach
back as much as possible with
your right leg; reach forward with
both arms.

⊙ Position the waist down, but your
head and chest up.

⊙ Keep your standing leg straight
and try to find the seesaw point.

⊙ Feel your body stretching in all
directions and imagine the muscles
wrapping around the bones.

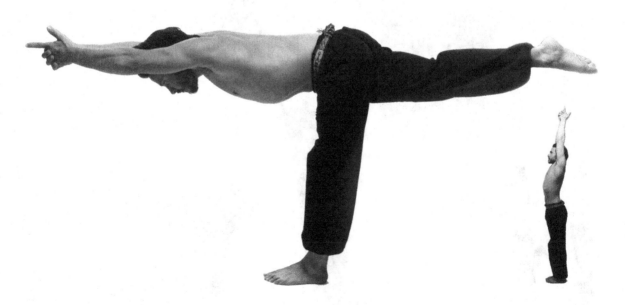

8. Groin Stretch

Open your legs wide, keeping your feet parallel. Stretch your arms over your head and then open them to the sides. With the palms facing forward, hinge at the waist and fold down. Grab your heels and try to bring your forehead to the floor.

Fig. 9.8: Groin Stretch

- Keep eyes focused on the floor.

- Pull yourself down by bending your elbows and using the biceps.

- Keep your legs locked and make sure that your pelvis is symmetrical.

- Keep your brow relaxed.

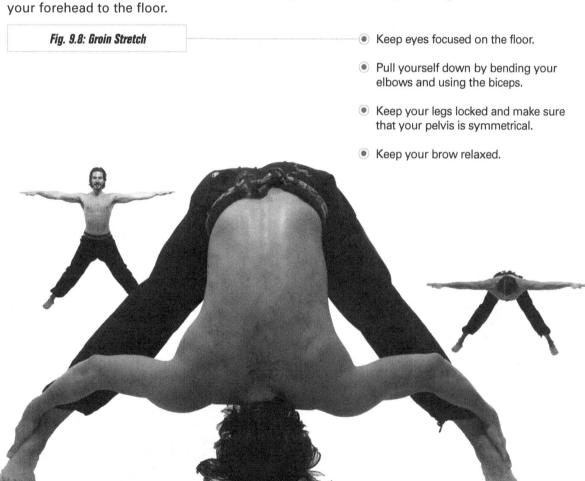

9. Side-Angle Pose

Return to center and reach your arms over your head to stretch. Open your legs a few feet apart, feet parallel. Turn the left heel in so it lines up with the arch of the right foot. Bring your hands to your sides and open your shoulders as wide as possible, facing forward. Finally, sit into the left leg, keeping your opposite knee joint straight. Bend your body and lower your left hand down to the earth, fingers together and pointed. Lift your right arm to the sky.

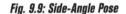

Fig. 9.9: Side-Angle Pose

- Lengthen the spine as you reach your hand down to the floor.

- Bring your chin to your upper shoulder and your eyes to the sky.

- Rotate your chest up.

- Continue to maintain energy through both arms. The hand that is down should bear little weight.

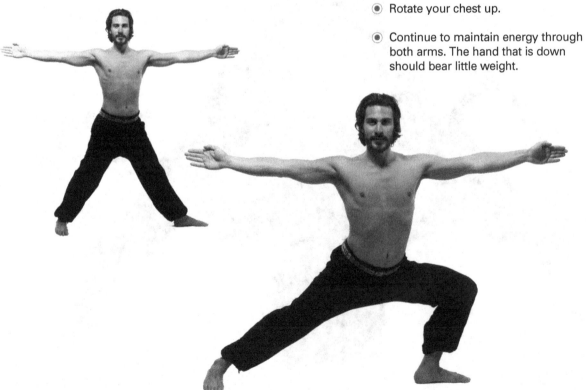

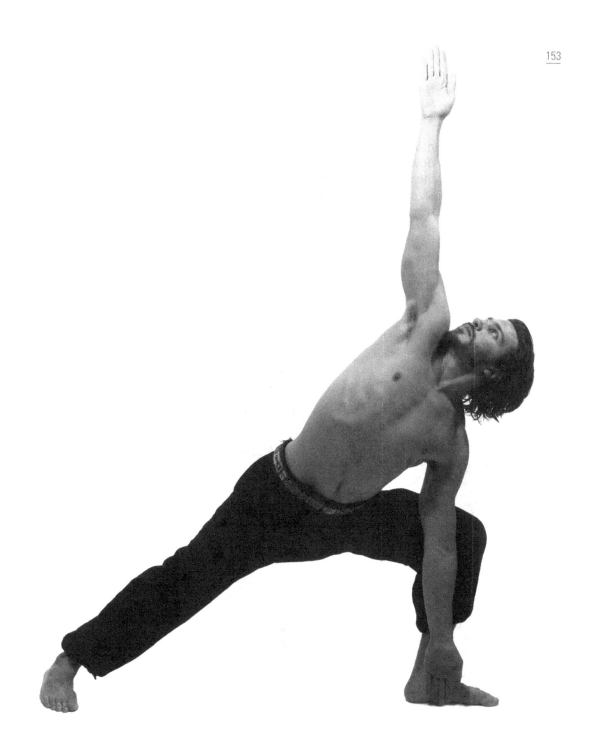

INVERSIONS

The following postures are excellent for decompressing the spine and working on strength and balance. They are said to improve concentration and brain function, because they bring added blood to the head; also the postures are supposed to enliven the pituitary, pineal, and thymus glands. These postures should be practiced against a wall or with a spotter in the beginning. Generally women should not practice these postures during their menstrual cycles, as prolonged inversion may disrupt the flow of blood, though I know many yoginis (female yogis) who continue to practice every day, and just hold the postures for less time.

10. Handstand

Find a flat wall to practice against. Loosen your wrists. Facing the wall, place your hands down about six inches from it and, with one leg straight and the other following behind, try to kick up. When you have both legs up, squeeze your abs and push the floor with your hands. Point your feet and squeeze both legs together. Beginners can practice doing cartwheels in order to get the feeling of going up on the hands.

Fig. 9.10: Handstand

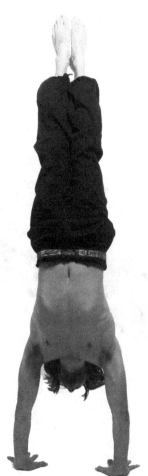

- ◉ Keep the belly tucked.

- ◉ Push the floor.

- ◉ Try to reach for the ceiling with the legs.

- ◉ Push the floor with the hands.

- ◉ Extend through your shoulders and squeeze your legs together.

11. Headstand

Contrary to popular belief, the headstand doesn't compress the spine in a negative way; when practiced correctly, it leads to weightlessness and buoyancy. The trick to safe and effective headstands is to push the floor. In order to do so, the head and neck must be properly aligned so you are pushing evenly through the entire skull. When the head is aligned properly, the weight of the body loads evenly through all the vertebrae, but when it is improperly aligned, the weight compounds wherever there is a weakness. It is absolutely essential that you keep your neck long and push through the top of your head!

Fold your mat twice so that it is extra thick and place it on the floor against a flat wall. Sit gently on your knees in front of it. Lean forward and place your forearms on the mat, lacing your fingers together. Open your elbows shoulder width. Place your head down on the mat, inside the boundary of your hands, pushing directly through the top of the head, and slightly to the front. Your hands are now behind your head. Press up off your knees, straightening your legs, and walk toward your head with your feet. You are now in a downward dog position—except your head is on the mat. When you can't walk any closer, bend one leg in and then the other.

Try to balance in this position. Straighten one leg up to the ceiling, and then straighten the other leg. Balance here, continuing to push through the top of the head, with your neck straight. When you are ready, lower your feet by bending them into the chest and then to the floor. Rest. After the headstand, lie flat on the back and rest for a few moments.

Be sure to breathe and control any fears. ◉

If you feel strain in the neck, come down immediately. ◉

To avoid strain, push directly though the top of the head. ◉

Use the wall only for balance; try not to lean on it. ◉

Keep your abs tight and reach for the ceiling with your feet. ◉

There should be one line from your feet—to knees to hip to head. ◉

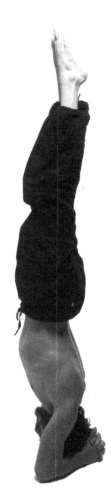

Fig. 9.11: Headstand

12. Plough II (see fig. 7.1.4 for a beginner's level)

From the relaxation position, kick your legs over your head and lengthen out the neck. Reach your arms behind you and lace your fingers together. Stretch your legs as much as possible, but be careful not to over-stretch the neck. Try to place your knees on either side of your ears and your hands down to the floor. Slowly roll down, vertebra by vertebra for final relaxation, or go directly into shoulder stand.

Fig. 9.12: Plough

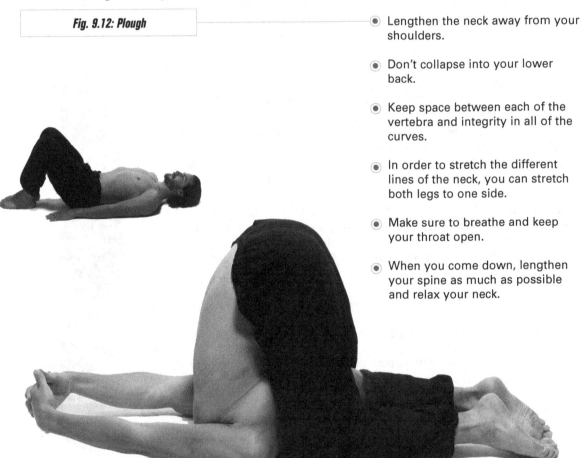

- Lengthen the neck away from your shoulders.

- Don't collapse into your lower back.

- Keep space between each of the vertebra and integrity in all of the curves.

- In order to stretch the different lines of the neck, you can stretch both legs to one side.

- Make sure to breathe and keep your throat open.

- When you come down, lengthen your spine as much as possible and relax your neck.

13. Shoulder Stand

Return to the plough pose (fig. 9.12), kicking your legs over your head, lacing your fingers, and straightening out your arms. Make sure to create space for your neck and continue to breathe normally. (You may need to rotate the shoulder blades down and back to create a good resting platform. This can be accomplished by rocking from side to side.) Bend your elbows and place your palms on your back ribcage, as close to your shoulder blades as possible. Bend your knees into your chest, making sure your weight is over your shoulders. In the same manner as the headstand, slowly straighten your legs upward. Reach for the sky with your feet. After ten to twenty breaths, roll back down, lowering the body vertebra by vertebra. Rest in the dead body (corpse pose) position. After completing the shoulder stand, it is advisable to rest for a while and then do some light extension of the neck. Traditionally the shoulder stand is followed by the "fish," which involves resting on the back and then arching the chest upwards and resting on the top of the head. I have left it out here, as it can put excessive compression on the vertebrae of the neck.

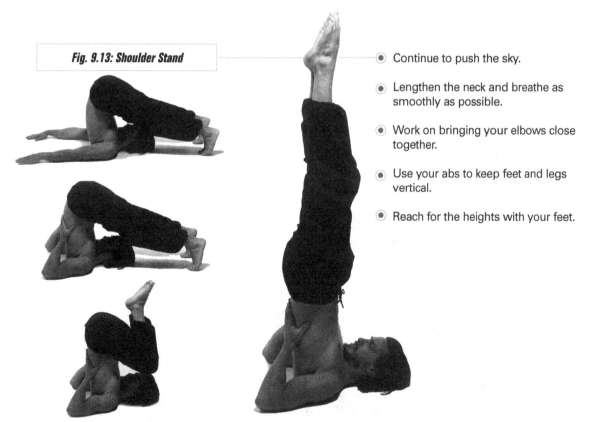

Fig. 9.13: Shoulder Stand

- Continue to push the sky.

- Lengthen the neck and breathe as smoothly as possible.

- Work on bringing your elbows close together.

- Use your abs to keep feet and legs vertical.

- Reach for the heights with your feet.

SEATED POSES

The following is a sampling of postures to be performed on a mat or a blanket. Begin in the dead body position and stretch the body long; then roll up quickly and stretch forward for a forward bend.

14. Forward Bend (seated)

Sit with your legs out in front of you, lift your chest and your arms, and reach to the sky. Bend and lengthen your body forward, feeling the stretch in your pelvis. Grab your two big toes with your thumb and forefinger and straighten your legs. Flex your feet, pulling your toes toward you, and bring your elbows down, trying to touch the ground with them. Work on folding completely flat, bringing your forehead to your shins, your chest to your knees and your abdomen to your thigh. In this position, you can practice being active and also being passive, alternately stretching hard and resting.

Fig. 9.14: Forward Bend

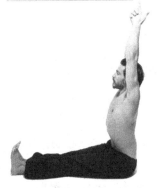

- ◉ Use advancement breathing to maintain your effort.

- ◉ Try to keep your legs straight.

- ◉ Feel the energy moving in both directions.

- ◉ Bring your feet and toes toward you.

- ◉ Push through the heels.

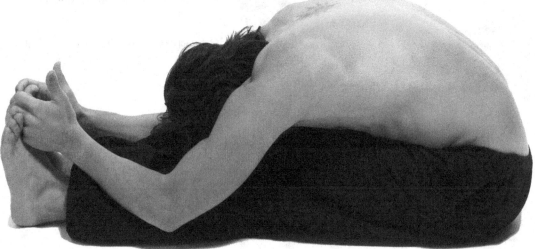

15. Camel

Turn over and sit on your heels. Rise up onto your knees and reach back with your hands on the butt. Lower one hand down and then the other so that both hands are resting on your heels. Bring your head back to look at the wall behind you and bring your hips forward, engaging your abs. For a mellower version, you can lift your feet so that you are on the toes, now the heels will be a few inches higher.

Fig. 9.15: Camel

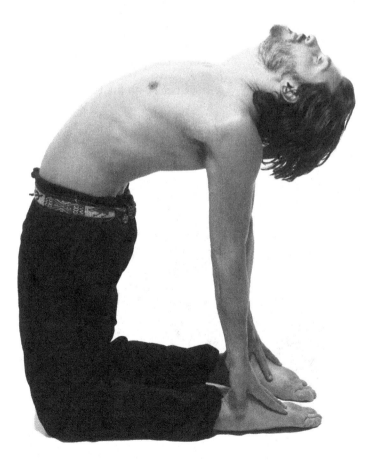

- Push forward from the hip.

- Make sure your knees and feet are even.

- Arch all the way back before you drop your head down.

- Keep your brow relaxed as you look for the wall.

- Don't forget to breathe.

- After finishing the camel, stretch forward in child's pose (see fig. 9.16a) to release your lower back.

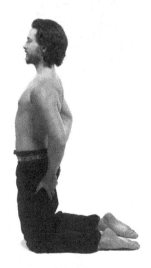

16. Bow

Lie on the mat so you are resting on your stomach (there are a lot of postures in this position, but some are covered by the Pilates or Sun Salute chapters). Reach back with your right arm and grab the outside of your right foot, then your left arm to your left foot. Arch up and kick back simultaneously to stretch the spine. Breathe into the spaces between your vertebrae. When you are finished, sit back on your heels and stretch your arms forward (child's pose; see fig. 9.16a), then come up to a seated position.

Fig. 9.16: Bow

Fig. 9.16a: Childs' Pose

⦿ Keep your toes together.

⦿ Keep your brow relaxed but look for the ceiling.

⦿ Keep the center of gravity over your abdomen.

⦿ Kick back with the legs.

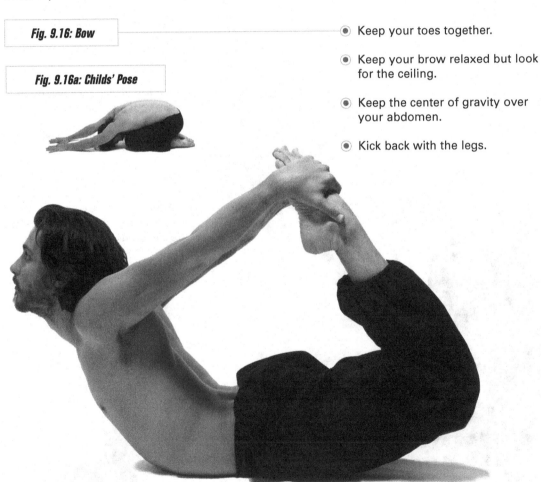

17. Spinal Twist

From a seated position, cross your right leg over the left so that your right foot (on your crossed leg) is adjacent to the left knee. Inhale and lift your lower back/ribcage, and then rotate across your raised knee. Exhale. Place your left hand outside your right knee and use the other arm to lift you up. Try to stay in position. Turn and look over the shoulder. Come back to neutral and repeat on the other side..

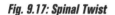

Fig. 9.17: Spinal Twist

- Keep your lower back lifted and turn your ribcage as much as possible.

- Try to keep both hips on the mat.

- After holding the pose, reach behind your back with your arms. Try to open the chest as you look up and behind you.

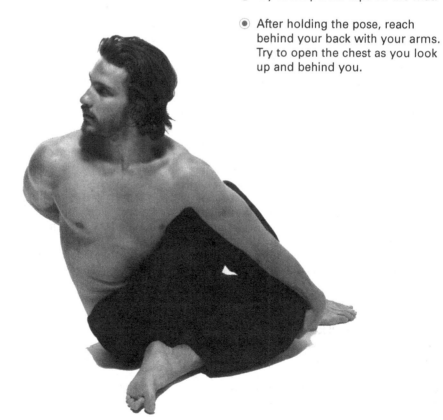

DAILY PRACTICE

This hatha yoga practice can be executed from start to finish, or in your own desired sequences. A good sequence is to do the following asanas every night: four sun salutes, the tree, the forward bend, the camel, the headstand, the shoulder stand, the plough, the bow, and the spinal twist. End with the dead body for a ten-minute relaxation period.

Yoga is a bit of a paradox. By mastering your body, it teaches you to free yourself of the burden of body; it teaches you how to apply effort with noneffort. Don't force yourself, but apply constant energy. As the saying goes, *the only way out is through.* These exercises are meant to release your mind from its confinement in the five senses (the body's perspective). They teach you to go beyond to the sixth sense of the mind, in order to find the strength and poise to endure whatever life throws at us. The stretches can also unlock hidden memories and subconscious elements.

This body is not *you*, you are the Atman, the individual spark of the great Brahman—the ultimate impersonal reality underlying everything in the universe, from which everything comes and everything returns. *Moksha* or liberation is the realization that the world is but an illusion, a mortal screen behind which the immortal energies dance. These immortal energies, in the form of thought and creative intention, organize the world around us. You create your own reality. You are the master of your body. It is all in the power of your mind.

THE PRINCIPLES OF EFFICIENCY

What follows are key concepts, thoughts, and meditations to help you get the most from the exercises in this book and, specifically, the Advancement Set. As you progress, and especially if you become a teacher, it is important to understand your body in terms of meta-concepts—universal qualities.

Dynamic tension.

Many of these exercises work because of dynamic tension—the process of engaging and releasing certain muscles. The principles of *yang* and *yin*, or activity and receptivity, are critical for understanding efficient movement. Mostly, the arms and the legs work under these rules. For example, as the biceps engage, the triceps must release, and vice versa. This is critical. When opposing muscle groups fail to release, it is known as *antagonistic tension*. This can work for or against you. If it is unconscious, it limits you; used consciously, it provides power and elasticity. The key is to learn to contract certain muscles in the core (core strength) in order to maximize the strength and stability of the limbs. Remember, efficient movement involves not just turning muscles on, but also turning muscles off. You must bring equal awareness to contraction and relaxation, in the same way that a guitar is tuned by turning some strings tighter and some looser.

We are designed symmetrically, but life is asymmetrical.

Part of what makes the language of the body simple is that we are designed symmetrically. If you understand one arm, you understand the other one. One of the main goals of Integrated Exercise is to restore balance to an asymmetrical world. As we practice, we learn to stay centered and use our limbs in the best way possible, which is to say, balanced and symmetrically.

Space is grace.

Another key to power and weightlessness is having space in the joint. A joint is the articulation of two or more bones (elbow joint and wrist joint, for example). When the joint is compressed, it lacks lubrication. When it is expanded, but not too much, it glides on pure magnetism, the invincible force of chi.

Synergistic curves.
A guitarist checks the tune of each of her six strings. Then she compares the strings to each other. A proper chord can only be attained when all the strings are vibrating in harmony. Similarly, integrated movement is achieved when various moving parts of the body are coordinated. When this happens, the whole is truly greater than the sum of its parts, and high levels of power and flexibility can be achieved.

The spine has three main curves, the lumbar (lower back), the thoracic (middle back), and the cervical (neck). If any one of these curves is out of place, it will negatively impact the entire spine. When they are all aligned, true power is unleashed.

Law of repeating patterns.
The design of the human body is so simple and efficient that certain patterns are repeated. Similarly, when you learn a few basic ideas or principles, you can apply them universally.

Subtle movement.
Meditative movement is a great way to gain understanding and decipher coded messages from your physique. You can lie on your back and do micro-movements—small, slow rotations. Where does the joint catch? Where is the circle interrupted? Revelation is born from this subtle awareness.

Muscles pull way better than they push.
It is important to remember that muscles pull better than they push. When I am doing a biceps curl, it is the biceps pulling the weight, not the triceps pushing the weight up. When the triceps refuses to let go, it leads to drag. When muscles are unconsciously engaged to push, they experience stress and misalignment. For example, many people literally lean back on their spines. This causes the muscles to compress and work harder to hold up the body.

Isometric contraction.
There are times when muscles stabilize from underneath without mobilizing the joint. This elongated motion is called Isometric contraction. This form of contraction is used by the core muscles during push-ups, and in the extended positions of yoga.

Moving by degrees.
Going from relaxation to full contraction is a high-speed, rapid motion and can cause joint pain and discomfort. One of the keys to tuning the body is awareness of partial contraction—of only using the necessary force to execute a task. Moving by degrees means that instead of contracting directly from 1–10, you go through every gear: 1, 2, 3, 4, 5 … 10. This minimizes compression and friction in a joint.

The circle of ease.
Every joint has a comfortable range of motion. The goal of Integrated Exercise is to safely increase the boundaries by challenging strength and range of motion simultaneously. This can only be achieved by remaining in the circle of ease. When you move outside of this zone, you increase the wear and tear on the joint and decrease efficiency. Inside the efficiency zone, muscles seem to last forever, because there is very little friction in the joint.

Chapter 10. *Pilates Style Exercises*

In the past twenty years, Pilates has made a surge into the spotlight of modern exercise. There is one simple reason: It works. Pilates was developed by Joseph Pilates, who combined elements of classic yoga with Western gymnastics and physical therapy. The result is an extremely effective system of total body unification.

What he developed was a science of control with the power to transform posture, heal injuries, and improve strength and range of motion. Pilates was in fact the first modern exercise synthesis, and it worked according to many of the same principles as Integrated Exercise.

After his death, Joseph Pilates left behind a direct lineage of followers. Devout disciples practice the Pilates method, and the name is trademarked to denote a specific sequence of exercises. Indeed, this school maintains high integrity and puts its teachers through a rigorous training program.

You can't patent a single exercise, and so the ideas and genius of Pilates have proliferated. Predictably, the integrity varies with the splinter schools; look for a teacher who embodies qualities of grace and mastery and who communicates effectively. *A good teacher will be calm, thorough, and vigilant about your safety.*

Pilates training is a great complement to the exercises in this book, and so it is recommended that you seek out a certified Pilates center in your area. You will discover a wealth of exercises both on the floor (mat work) and on various machines, including the Reformer, the Wonder Chair, and the Cadillac.

In order to master the more difficult yoga postures, you need to boost and refine your quality of movement. Pilates training emphasizes core strength and the distribution of that power to the limbs. It also focuses on the recruitment of the lats (*latisimus dorsi*) muscles. These are the long muscles on the side of the body that essentially connect the core strength to the arms. Your lats can also be used to support the arms from underneath. Unlike yoga, Pilates exercises do not hyperextend the shoulders or neck, and so it can be a good way to relax and release after a strenuous yoga practice. The lat muscles are recruited to keep the shoulders down and wide. The emphasis is on turning off the traps (*trapezius*) and pecs (*pectorals*) in exchange for more deltoid and lat firing.

What follows are Pilates-style exercises for the abs, back, and hips. These sets will help you to further strengthen your core and improve your functional range of motion. You can use each part of this chapter separately, as a complement to the rest of the book, or you can do the entire set of exercises, which will give you a solid half-hour Pilates workout.

TIPS FOR THE PILATES WORKOUT

With most of these exercises, there are variations for heavy, medium, and light approaches. In general, I have presented the medium exercises. To make an abdominal exercise harder, lower your legs more; to make it easier, raise your legs toward the ceiling. For leg exercises, a bent knee will lessen the difficulty. Always bend your knees into the chest before lowering them down to the floor. Try to keep your shoulders relaxed, and release your neck whenever it is tense. People with neck pain should support the head with a pillow. Use the breath to squeeze your abs, and try to make every exercise count. Put your full mind and body intention into each movement, and don't let yourself defer to habitual patterns. A good Pilates teacher will make all of this clear, but if you decide to practice on your own, it will be your responsibility. Again, these exercises are presented from the point of view of Integrated Exercise and may differ slightly from traditional Pilates. Either way, go slow and be thorough. Safety first.

1. BASIC ELEMENTS—THE CORE

All Pilates-style exercises emanate from these basic elements that establish the way you use your breath and awareness of your core. Seat yourself on the mat and lower yourself into a supine position (on your back). The basics are all done from this position.

1.1. Forced Exhalation

Bend your knees slightly, contract your abs, and find the pelvic position that will engage your abs and relax your lower back, or you can opt for a natural curve, what is called the neutral spine. Inhale. Feel your ribs connect to your pelvis. Then on the exhalation, curl your head up and place your hands on your belly—feel the contraction in your abdominals. These exercises are no exception to any others in this book ... breath is the key. You should use the breath to work your abs as if you are wringing water out of a towel. When you think you are empty, squeeze some more.

If your ribs come up as in this picture, engage your abs and muscles of the pelvic floor to anchor the ribcage.

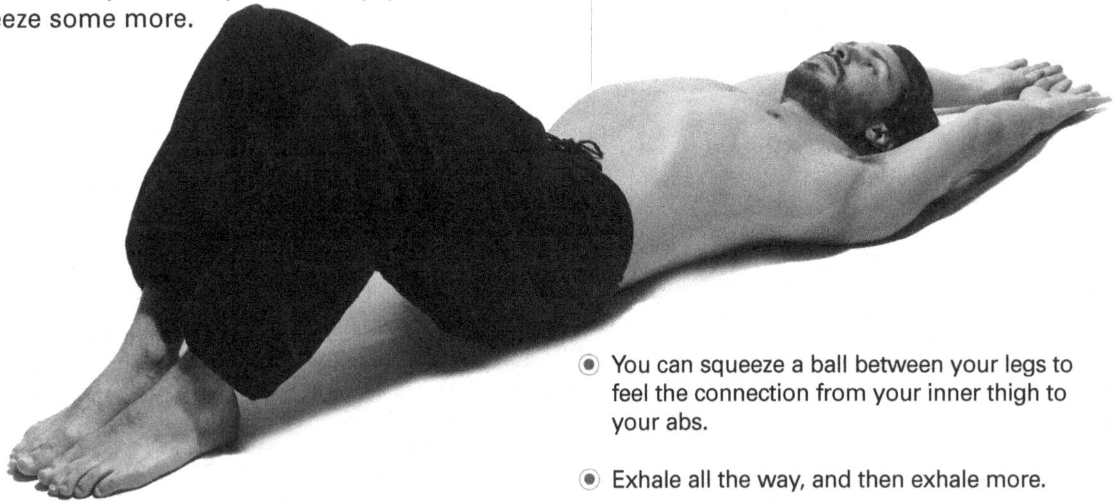

Fig. 10.1.1: Forced Exhalation

- You can squeeze a ball between your legs to feel the connection from your inner thigh to your abs.

- Exhale all the way, and then exhale more.

- Keep space between your chin and chest.

- Relax your jaw.

- Can you feel how your abdominals run all the way from your chest to your pubic bone?

1.2. Straight-Arm Crunch

Bend your knees slightly and place both feet on the floor. Lengthen both arms over your head and extend the energy through your fingertips (see fig.10.1.1). Engage the lat muscles and begin a slow exhalation. As you do so, lift your arms off the floor, keeping them straight. Continue raising them and when they pass over your head, begin to lift the head up, keeping the chin slightly tucked. Now begin to lower your arms all the way down to your sides, stopping them about two inches above the floor. At this point, you should be completely out of breath. Hold for a moment, and then inhale as your raise your arms back up. When they pass your eyes, lower the head down.

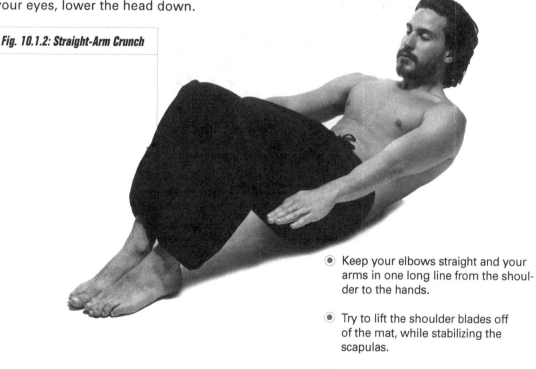

Fig. 10.1.2: Straight-Arm Crunch

- Keep your elbows straight and your arms in one long line from the shoulder to the hands.

- Try to lift the shoulder blades off of the mat, while stabilizing the scapulas.

- Keep your face relaxed.

- Rather than using momentum, simply glide up and down.

1.3. Single-Arm Crunch

With the feet in the same position,
lift one arm over your head and let
the other one rest by your side.
Repeat the previous exercise but
with only one arm at a time. Once
again, don't lift your head until your
hand has passed your eyes. As you
lift your upper body, begin to twist,
anchoring yourself with the opposite
hip; this will give you dynamic tension and ultra-burn. Then switch
arms. After completing the exercise,
bend both knees into the chest and
rest.

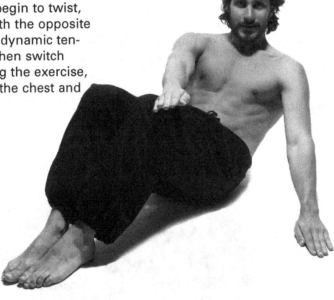

Fig. 10.1.3: Single-Arm Crunch

- As you twist, reach for the far corner of the room.

- Don't lift the hip as you turn.

- Lengthen the spine.

- Only bring your shoulders up three-quarters of the way.

1.4. Leg Extension

Inhale. Place your hands behind your head and touch your heels together, keeping the toes apart. Bring your knees up toward your chest and lift your head. While exhaling straighten your legs out forty-five degrees (ninety degrees for beginners) above the floor. Inhale them back into your chest and repeat. To finish, bend your knees into the chest, put your head back down, and rest.

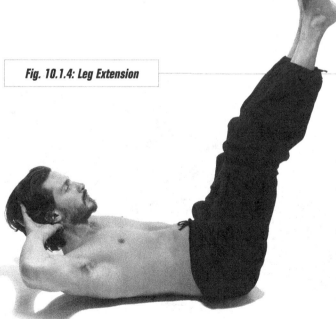

Fig. 10.1.4: Leg Extension

- ⦿ Keep energy in your legs as your straighten the knees.

- ⦿ Contract your belly to protect your lower back.

- ⦿ Keep your elbows wide.

- ⦿ Keep space between your chin and chest. Relax your jaw.

- ⦿ Try to lift your shoulder blades off the mat.

1.5. Single Leg Stretch

Bend both knees into the chest.
Place both hands two inches below
your right knee and lengthen your
left leg out six inches above the mat.
(Beginners or persons with knee
injuries can leave the head down,
bend the knee to ninety degrees,
and extend the other leg up to the
ceiling). Curl your head up and pull
the bent leg into your chest as you
contract the abs with the breath.
Inhale as you switch legs. Exhale as
you bring your left leg in.

- ⦿ Pull your knee straight into the chest, and maintain pelvic stability.

- ⦿ Keep energy in the extended leg.

- ⦿ Keep the elbows wide.

- ⦿ Use your biceps to pull, rather than the pectoral muscles.

Fig. 10.1.5: Single Leg Stretch

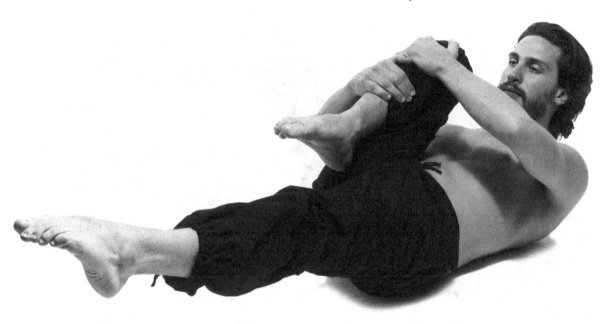

1.6. Elbow to Knee

Place both hands behind your head and keep your elbows wide. Lengthen the left leg and keep the right knee bent into your chest. On exhalation, lift your head up and twist, touching the left elbow to the right knee. Inhale; lower your upper body down and switch legs. Exhale as right elbow goes to left knee. To finish, bend both knees into your chest and squeeze.

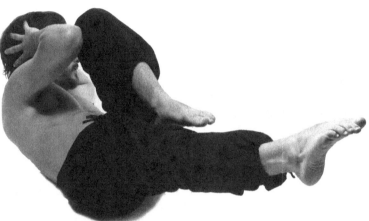

Fig. 10.1.6: Elbow to Knee

- Keep the elbows wide and the toes pointed.

- Turn from the ribcage, not from the shoulder, and try to maintain pelvic stability.

- Keep energy in the extended leg.

- Anchor the hips.

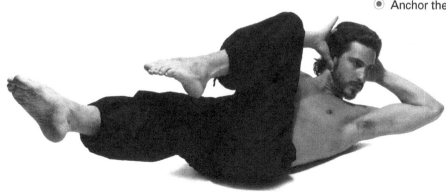

1.7. Scissors

Straighten one leg up to the ceiling and grab behind that knee. Reach the other leg away until it is six inches above the floor. Both legs should be straight. (Beginners can bend both knees and keep the foot at forty-five degrees above the floor). Curl your head up and pull with your biceps to move your straight leg toward your chest. Then switch.

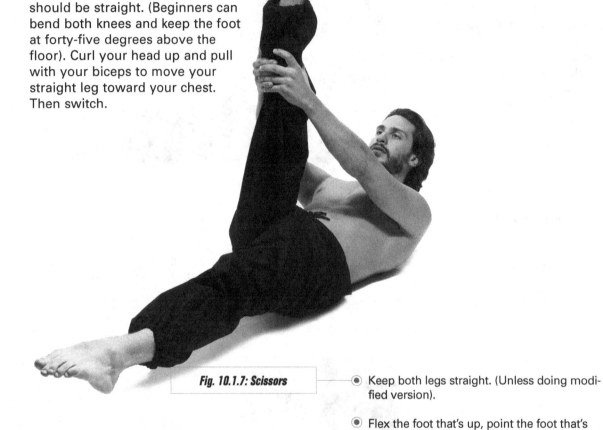

Fig. 10.1.7: Scissors

- Keep both legs straight. (Unless doing modified version).

- Flex the foot that's up, point the foot that's down.

- Inhale while legs are switching.

- Exhale to pull the leg in.

1.8. Hundreds

Straighten your knees, point your feet, and then lift both legs up to the ceiling. Hold the legs there—for a harder exercise, you can lower the legs to forty-five degrees. With your legs in either position, lengthen your arms over your head, engage the lats, and then float your arms up. When they pass your eyes, lift your head and start bringing your arms down until they are two inches above the floor. Then pump your arms up and down for up to 100 counts, breathing with rapid, forced exhalation. Don't allow your elbows to bend, and keep your hands straight.

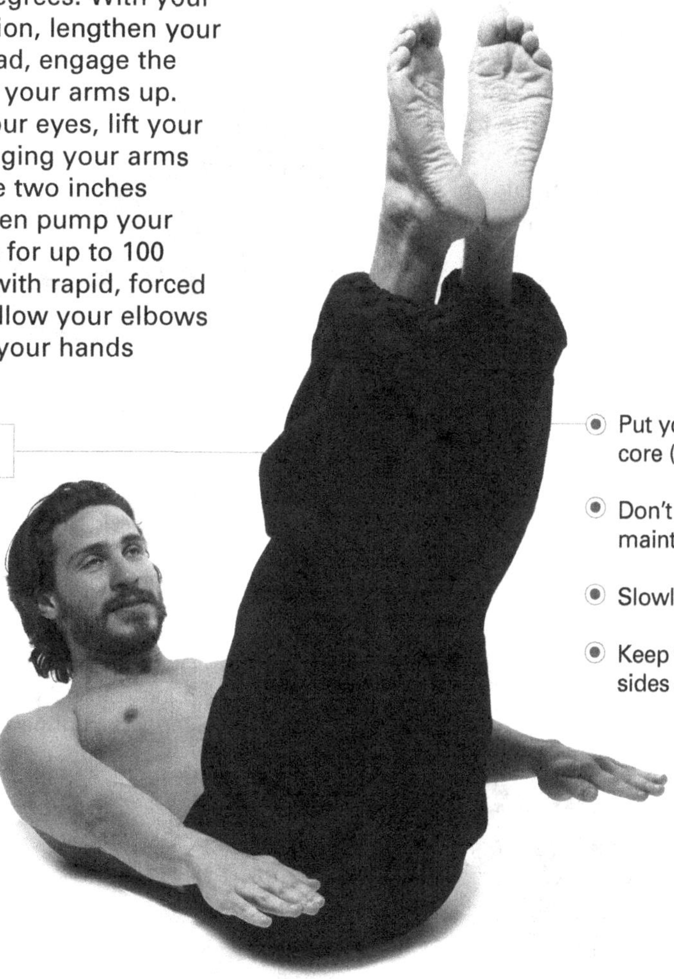

Fig. 10.1.8: Hundreds

- Put your awareness in your core (abdomen).

- Don't use momentum. Always maintain balance and control.

- Slowly lower yourself down.

- Keep your arms by your sides and your legs steady.

1.9. Roll-Up

Straighten both legs on the mat with your feet shoulder-width apart and your toes curled up. Reach your arms overhead, engage your lats, and stretch. On exhalation, float your arms past your eyes, lift your head, and then, using your core, lift your whole torso until you are sitting. Inhale when you are at the top and then exhale as you lean forward to stretch the hamstrings. Inhale back to sitting and then exhale slowly to lower yourself. Tuck. Tuck. Tuck. Lower yourself inch-by-inch until you are once again resting flat.

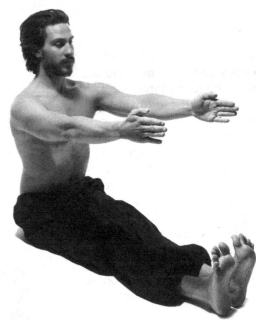

Fig. 10.1.9: Roll-Up

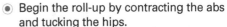 Lift your head when your hands pass your eyes.

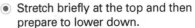 Begin the roll-up by contracting the abs and tucking the hips.

⊙ Stretch briefly at the top and then prepare to lower down.

⊙ On the way back down, continuously bring your belly button into your spine and tuck your pelvis.

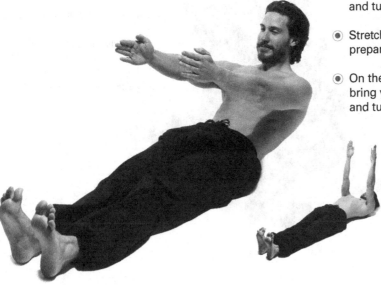

1.10 Roll-Up Twist

Lengthen one arm over your head and let the other one rest at your side. Keep your legs straight and your toes up as before. On exhalation, roll up slowly and reach your raised arm across your body and up. Try to keep the opposite hip anchored down and the ribs and pelvis connected.

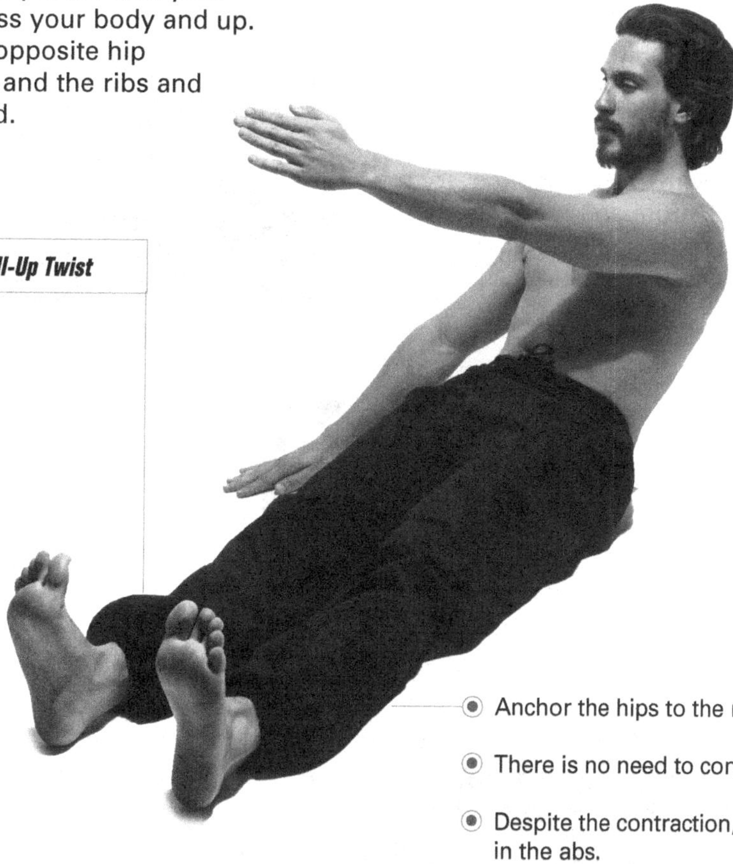

Fig. 10.1.10: Roll-Up Twist

- Anchor the hips to the mat.

- There is no need to come up all the way.

- Despite the contraction, try to keep length in the abs.

- As you breathe out, imagine that you are wringing water out of a towel, by squeezing your abs.

1.11. Pelvic Mobilization

Sit up and bend your legs into a butterfly position (soles of the feet together, knees apart). Reach in front of you and loosely lace your fingers, forming a circle with your arms. Slowly, inhale and lift your lower back and tuck your belly. This is back extension. Exhale as you begin to tuck back about six inches, rounding your lower back, and keeping the muscles of the pelvic floor active. Lift again, then tuck again, repeating the move ten times. With each repetition, try to lift the lower back more and more, so that you are mobilizing the spine and pelvis through flexion and extension.

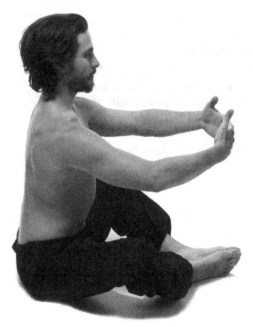

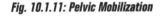
Fig. 10.1.11: Pelvic Mobilization

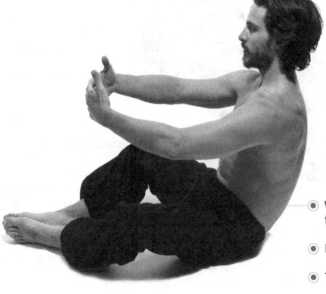

◉ With the back straight, bring your torso in front of the midline.

◉ Don't allow your lower back to pop out.

◉ Try to keep the spinal curves in harmony.

◉ Keep the legs symmetrical.

1.12. Saw

Straighten out your legs flat on the mat and spread them wide. Lift your lower back and open your arms into a wide T. Relax your shoulders and chest so the energy flows through your fingertips. Inhale. On exhalation, stretch forward and twist your torso and arm to reach the right hand past the left ankle. Inhale up to center and twist to the other side.

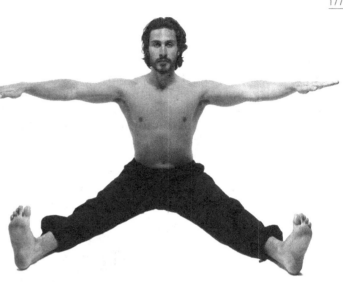

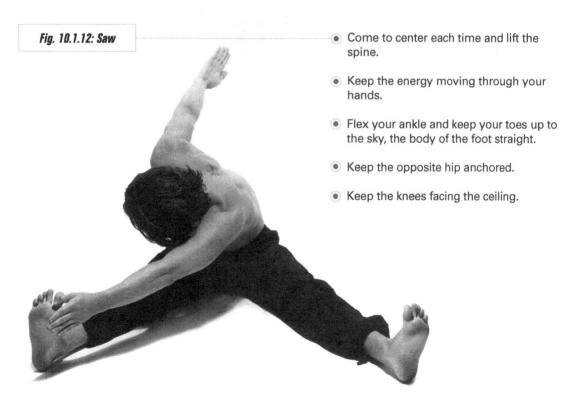

Fig. 10.1.12: Saw

- Come to center each time and lift the spine.

- Keep the energy moving through your hands.

- Flex your ankle and keep your toes up to the sky, the body of the foot straight.

- Keep the opposite hip anchored.

- Keep the knees facing the ceiling.

2. BACK EXTENSION

After you have completed the abdominal exercises, you should feel a good burn. The final exercise in the previous set was designed to stretch the lower back and increase hamstring flexibility. A healthy back is the result of balance between the abdominals and the lower back muscles. The following exercises are performed in a prone position (on your front). This sequence will help you combat the effects of age and stress, and balance the curves of your back by teaching you to arch your back (back extension), while maintaining stability in the shoulders. Be aware of over-contraction in the lower back and try to distribute the energy evenly. Feel the contraction (energy) in the entire length of the muscle, from the neck all the way to the tailbone. Aside from the stretches, each exercise should be performed ten times.

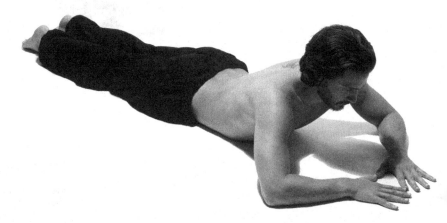

2.1. Quad Stretch

Lie on your stomach with your head to one side. Reach back and grab your right ankle with your right arm and stretch. Pull the leg in and push your pelvis into the mat so that you feel the center of the stretch in your upper quads. Hold for ten seconds; then switch sides. Again, if you have a knee injury don't go past ninety degrees.

Fig. 10.2.1: Quad Stretch

⊙ Push the pelvis into the floor.

⊙ Lengthen the lower back and focus the stretch on the front of the quad.

⊙ Keep the knees on the midline.

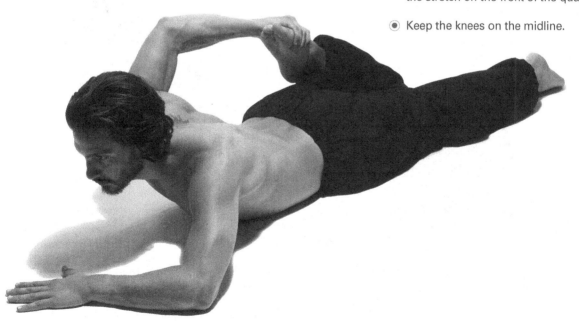

2.2. Single Leg Lift

Lower your leg and place your hands on the mat just beyond your head; make a diamond shape with the thumbs and forefingers touching. Bring awareness to your legs and imagine there is a laser pointing out through both your feet. Reach the feet away and feel the smooth contraction from your buttocks all the way to the tip of your toes. Now, lift and lower one leg, and then the other.

Fig. 10.2.2: Single Leg Lift

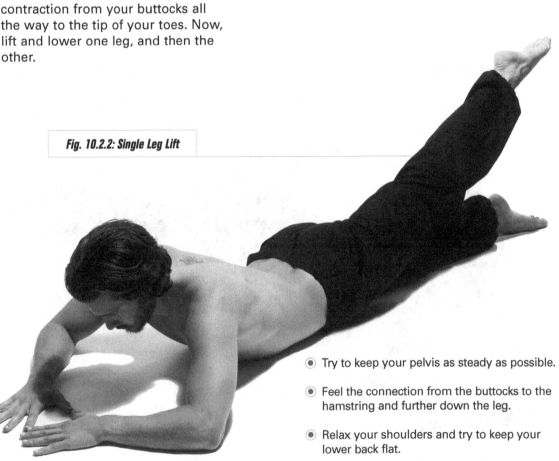

- Try to keep your pelvis as steady as possible.

- Feel the connection from the buttocks to the hamstring and further down the leg.

- Relax your shoulders and try to keep your lower back flat.

2.3. Double Leg Lift

In the same position, lift *both* legs
six inches off of the mat. Breathe.
Repeat.

Fig. 10.2.3: Double Leg Lift

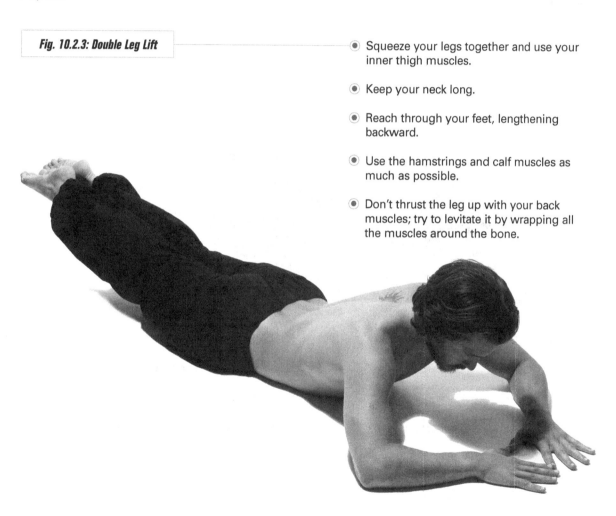

- Squeeze your legs together and use your inner thigh muscles.

- Keep your neck long.

- Reach through your feet, lengthening backward.

- Use the hamstrings and calf muscles as much as possible.

- Don't thrust the leg up with your back muscles; try to levitate it by wrapping all the muscles around the bone.

2.4. Open and Close the Legs

Still in the same position, use your lower back and buttocks to lift your legs; then open and close them ten times. Breathe. Rest.

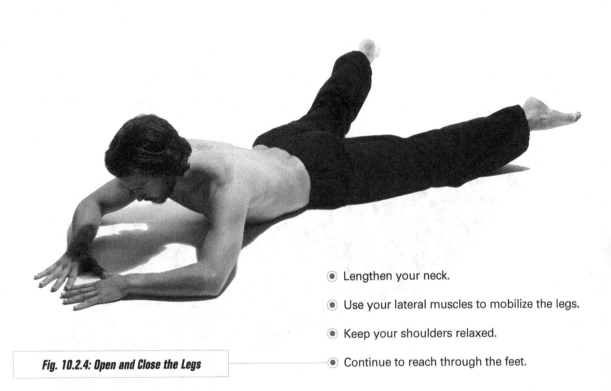

● Lengthen your neck.

● Use your lateral muscles to mobilize the legs.

● Keep your shoulders relaxed.

● Continue to reach through the feet.

Fig. 10.2.4: Open and Close the Legs

2.5. Upside Down Snow Angel

Reach the arms in front of you and place the palms together in prayer position. Straighten the elbows and put energy in the hands. On exhalation, lift the arms a few inches off of the floor and open them wide; follow through until the hands are by the side of the hip and then repeat. As the arms lift, the body will also lift, so that the upper part of the chest is off the mat. But make sure your shoulders stay away from the ears.

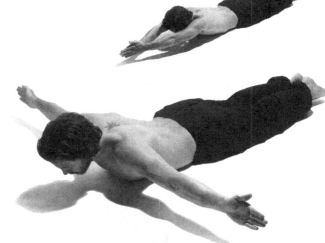

Fig. 10.2.5: Upside Down Snow Angel

- Keep your thumbs up.

- Lengthen through the neck, but don't hyperextend.

- Use your lat muscles to pull the arms close to your side.

- Try to extend in the middle of the back.

- Keep your shoulders wide.

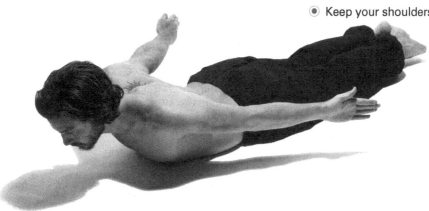

2.6. Swimming

With your arms straight and your palms down, bring both hands in front of you once again. Lift your head slightly and lengthen through the legs. Reach long and then lift one arm and the opposite leg. Alternate. To increase the difficulty, keep all the limbs off the floor and flutter as if you are swimming. Repeat for twenty counts.

Fig. 10. 2.6: Swimming

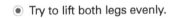

◉ Try to lift both legs evenly.

◉ Balance on the pelvis and try not to rock back and forth.

◉ Lengthen as much as possible through the limbs.

◉ Keep your arms straight and use the deltoids more than the muscles of the chest.

◉ Again, keep the shoulders away from the ears.

2.7. Rest Position (Child's Pose)

Lying on your stomach, place your hands down just above your head and press up onto all fours. Keeping your head down, scoot back onto your heels and reach your arms in front, rounding out your lower back and relieving any tension that has accumulated.

Fig. 10.2.7: Rest Position (Child's Pose)

⦿ Reach through the arms and try to get your shoulders above and behind your ears.

⦿ Breathe.

⦿ Release.

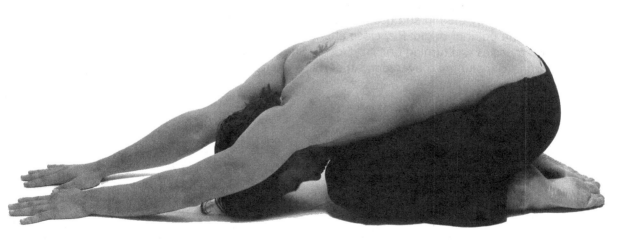

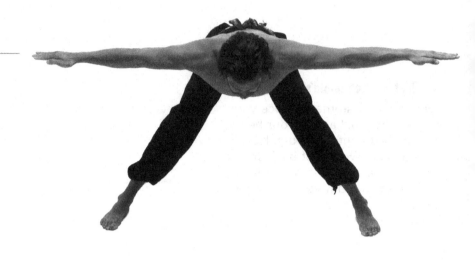

3. HIP FLEXIBILITY

This sequence is designed to enhance flexibility and range of motion in the hips and legs. It is important to learn to use the quads and the hamstrings to unstick the leg from the hip/pelvis. Maintain your focus for the duration of each exercise. Keep the spine and pelvis steady. The movement should come from the legs. Remember the idea of stabilizers and mobilizers? Here it is important to steady the hip and use the quads to mobilize. Feel your muscles moving all the way up from the point of origin. Pay close attention and try to find the circle of ease by turning off "grippy" muscles and turning on "lazy" ones. Start with small circles, and when you find the efficiency zone, expand the movement. All of these exercises are performed lying down on the mat.

3.1. Leg Lifts

Lie flat on your back and let your arms rest at your sides. Let the legs rest flat. On exhalation, lift one leg straight up to the ceiling. Keep your foot flexed and do not bend in the knee (unless doing modified version). Inhale and lower your leg down. Repeat ten times and then switch legs.

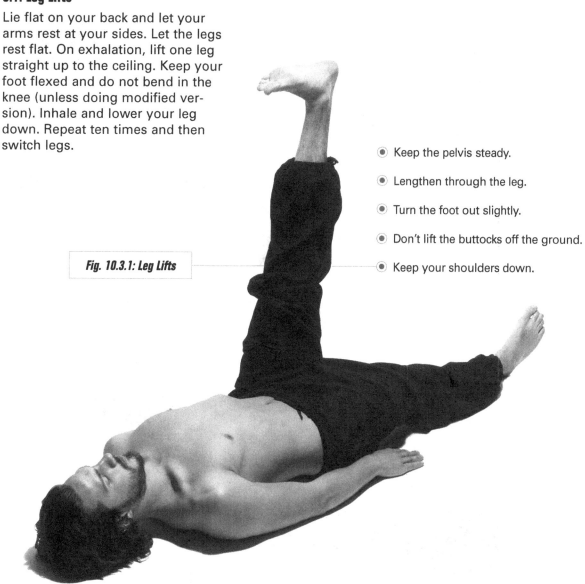

Fig. 10.3.1: Leg Lifts

- Keep the pelvis steady.
- Lengthen through the leg.
- Turn the foot out slightly.
- Don't lift the buttocks off the ground.
- Keep your shoulders down.

3.2. Leg Circles

In the same position and with the arms by your sides, lift your right leg up to the ceiling; point your foot and straighten the knee. Then, keeping the pelvis as steady as possible, begin to circle the whole leg. Imagine there is a beam of light emitted through your toes. Do ten circles in one direction, pause, and reverse. Switch legs and repeat the movements.

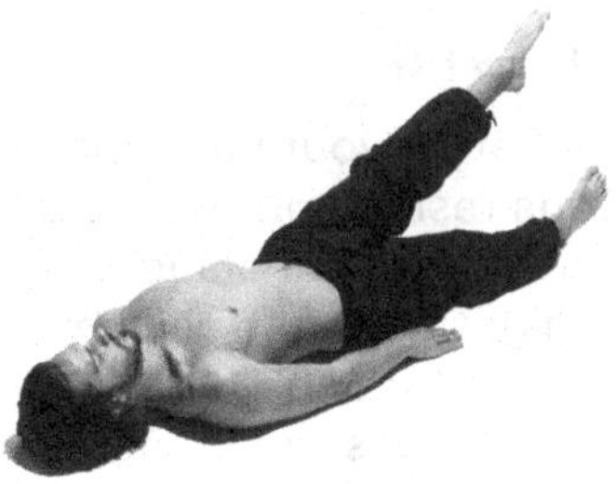

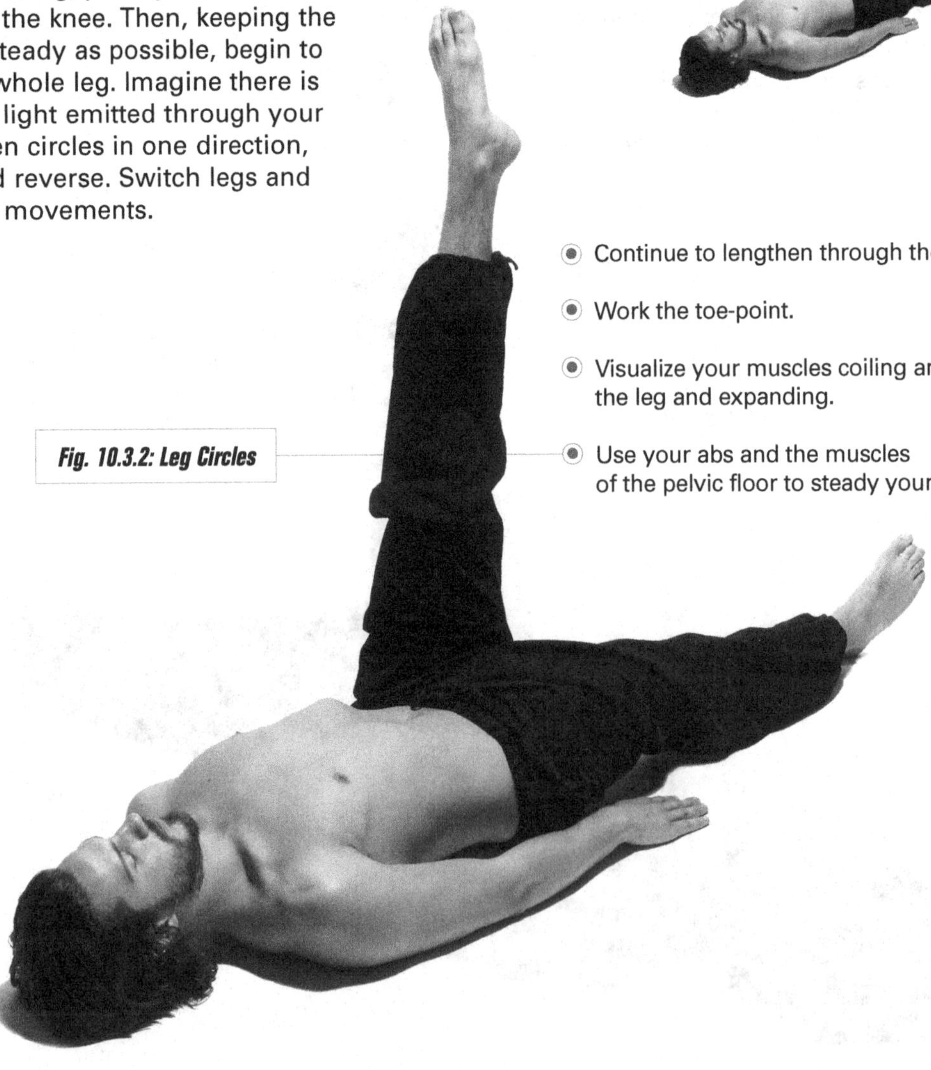

Fig. 10.3.2: Leg Circles

- Continue to lengthen through the leg.

- Work the toe-point.

- Visualize your muscles coiling around the leg and expanding.

- Use your abs and the muscles of the pelvic floor to steady your hip.

3.3. Working on Your Side

Roll over so you are lying on your side. Bend slightly at the waist. Rest your head in your the hand, supported by the elbow. Angle your bottom leg forward slightly and plant your foot. Then lift the top leg and bend the knee so that it is facing the ceiling. This is your position. You will switch to the other side and repeat each exercise with the other leg.

- Keep your elbow up.

- Lengthen through the neck.

- Don't let your pelvis tip.

- Keep the pelvis steady as you open the knee.

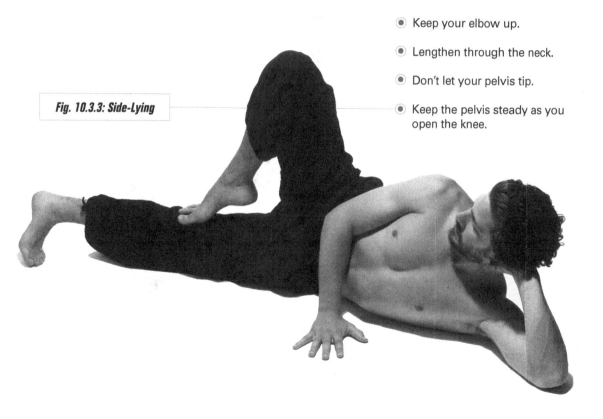

Fig. 10.3.3: Side-Lying

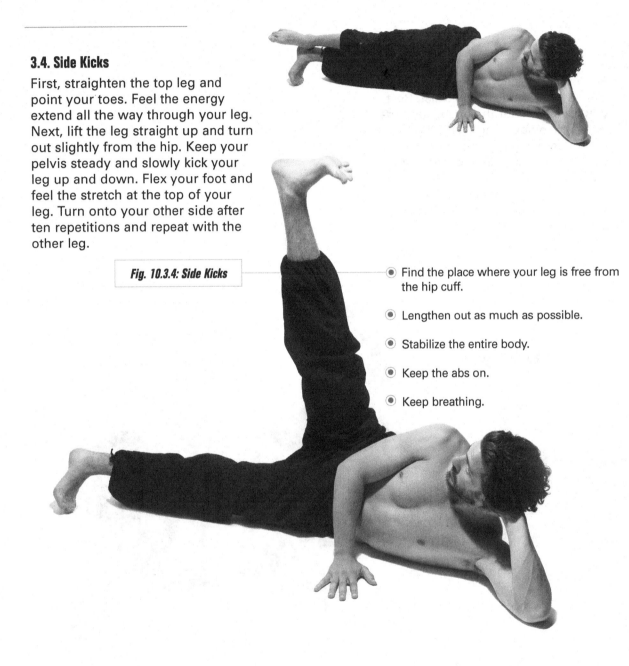

3.4. Side Kicks

First, straighten the top leg and point your toes. Feel the energy extend all the way through your leg. Next, lift the leg straight up and turn out slightly from the hip. Keep your pelvis steady and slowly kick your leg up and down. Flex your foot and feel the stretch at the top of your leg. Turn onto your other side after ten repetitions and repeat with the other leg.

Fig. 10.3.4: Side Kicks

- Find the place where your leg is free from the hip cuff.

- Lengthen out as much as possible.

- Stabilize the entire body.

- Keep the abs on.

- Keep breathing.

3.5. Hip Opener

In the same position, bend your top leg in until your toes are touching your opposite knee. Stabilize the pelvis and lift the leg straight. Try to maintain the turned out position in the thigh and flex the foot. When the leg is straight, pull it in for a stretch, and then lower it to the other heel. Keeping both legs straight, use your abs to lift both feet off the floor. Lower both legs and bend the top leg in again. Repeat ten times. Then turn over and switch legs.

Fig. 10.3.5: Hip Opener

- Keep your pelvis from tipping forward and back.

- Articulate from the hip.

- Keep your head steady, neck lengthened.

- Stretch your inner thigh.

- Work the buttocks.

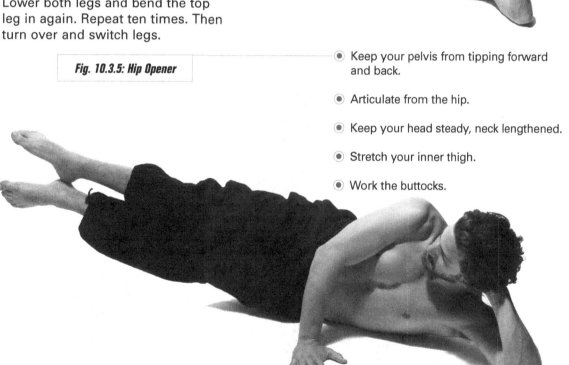

3.6. Sidewise Leg Circles

Maintain this position and straighten the leg to the ceiling. With maximal focus on pelvic stability, circle your leg. Begin small to feel for the circle of ease, and then gradually expand. You can do ten small and then ten large circles in each direction. Then turn over and repeat.

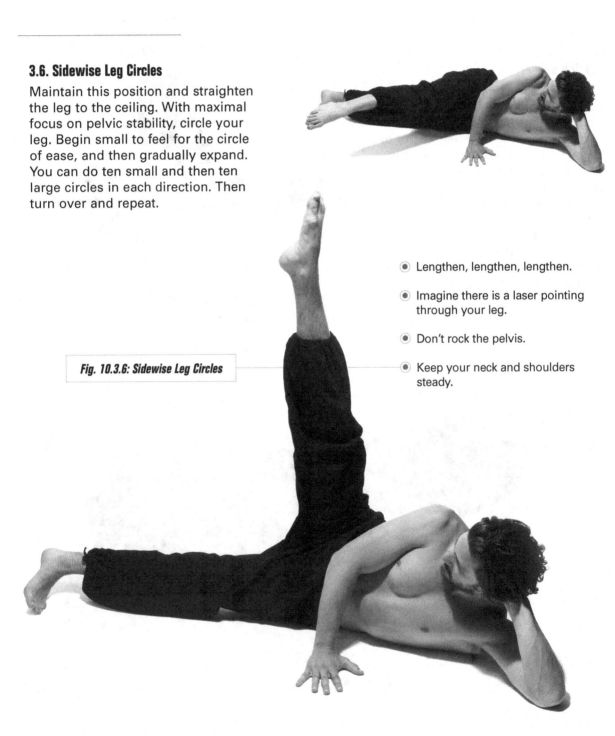

Fig. 10.3.6: Sidewise Leg Circles

- Lengthen, lengthen, lengthen.

- Imagine there is a laser pointing through your leg.

- Don't rock the pelvis.

- Keep your neck and shoulders steady.

COMPLETION

To complete this sequence, lie flat on your back and bend both knees in toward your chest. With your knees bent, slowly lower your feet to the floor and stretch your whole body. Roll over to one side and get up slowly. Walk slowly around the room. Feel the energy distribute evenly throughout your body. Feel your lower back release and your quads engage. Breathe naturally and notice the strength and elasticity in your abdomen. As you get up and walk away, try to keep your awareness in your core and your presence in your steps.

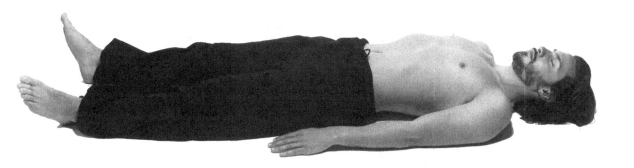

Chapter 11. *Martial Arts Exercises/ Basic Training*

Today's martial arts world owes much to the mind and work of Bruce Lee. Lee's martial prowess (as a fighter as opposed to an artist) is sometimes disputed, but his philosophical awareness and his film presence are undeniable. He trained his body in a universal way and sought to become like water—spontaneous, flowing, soft, yet powerful. He was also a pioneering integrated thinker who helped liberate the Chinese martial arts from the imperial stronghold that had imprisoned it. Lee was not confined by tradition, but he recognized the ancient disciplines as part of an ever-flowing river, an eternally renewed, bubbling, and creative source. This kind of thought is much aligned with Taoism, where the yin and yang—the pairs of opposites—are in an eternal confluence, and man must learn to become one with nature; he must learn to unite himself with its power. Bruce Lee's "style is no style" philosophy strived to overcome mental obstacles and rigid adherence to tradition in order to reach spontaneous and optimized instinct—the full expression of the human being. Lee systematized his learning into a new martial art, which he called the "way of the intercepting fist," or Jeet Kun Do (JKD) in Cantonese.

If you wish to learn the martial arts, you must learn to kick, punch, throw, and defend. In order to be successful at it, you must move with speed, efficiency, and grace. The most important elements are timing and the ability to learn and apply certain skills. A good fighter will use boxing or kung-fu techniques at a distance; throws, locks, and strikes in the medium range; and grappling as well as submission holds on the ground. The discipline must be studied as an integrated whole. And basic training can't be overlooked.

If you have no particular interest in martial applications, you will still find that learning to defend yourself helps improve awareness of your field of energy. These exercises refine the neuromuscular pathways of the limbs and help us learn to employ the creative skills of cadence, rhythm, and juking as we wrestle with life. Learning the art of self-defense improves your awareness of exactly where you are in time and space and how to flow seamlessly within that environment.

The martial arts exercises included in this chapter are also valuable to build strength; they cultivate not only the slow, controlled, flexible strength we have accomplished throughout this book, but also dynamic, explosive power.

The following exercises have been developed from various forms such as kung-fu, capoeira,* and gymnastics. They are not intended solely for their martial applications, but also for their training value. However, if you cultivate the qualities of the exercises, it will be easy to learn anything from Brazilian jujitsu to the Drunken Monkey. Once again, you will have a body that is ready to download all kinds of new software.

A Brazilian dance that incorporates martial arts movements.

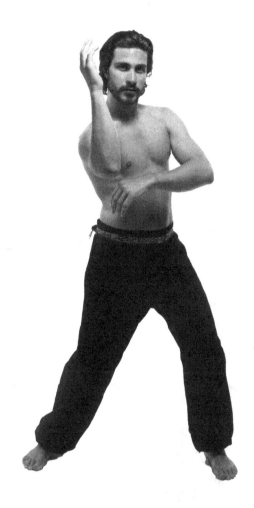

1. THE EIGHT GATES

The Eight Gates are extremely valuable for enhancing neurological awareness and timing. The Eight Gates refer to eight main areas of the body that must be defended, and they teach economy and efficiency of movement. You will learn to defend the upper, upper-middle, lower-middle, and lower parts of your body on both the right and left. The sequence offered here is my interpretation and is meant to be an exercise in efficiency and body awareness.

By quickly rotating the arms and the legs at the joint site, the hands and feet can defend more area in less time. This enhances body awareness by making you cognizant of how far you need to block—if you over-commit in your defense, you automatically leave yourself open. The quick rotation defends the desired area of your body but allows you to remain ready to defend the other parts, or to strike.

As you practice these exercises, bring your awareness to the edge of your energy field but try not to go beyond it. Keep the movements clean and gradually increase the tempo until you can move through the entire sequence rapidly and with fluid motion.

1.1. Horse Stance

To begin, stand with your feet slightly wider than your hips and sink down into the quads—the horse stance. Next, lift your arms up with your elbows bent and your hands just in front of your face.

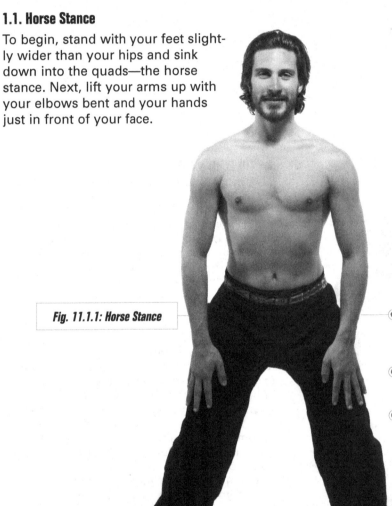

Fig. 11.1.1: Horse Stance

- Try to have a neutral spine (not overly tucked/extended) and allow the energy to sink into the earth.

- Root yourself and allow the power to come from your feet.

- Stand comfortably and relaxed.

1.2. Symmetrical Defense

With the arms by your face, become aware of the edges of your body and observe how a small motion of the hand is enough to make a precise block. Practice moving the hands a few inches in either direction. You can also move the head a little bit with a slight, serpentine motion.

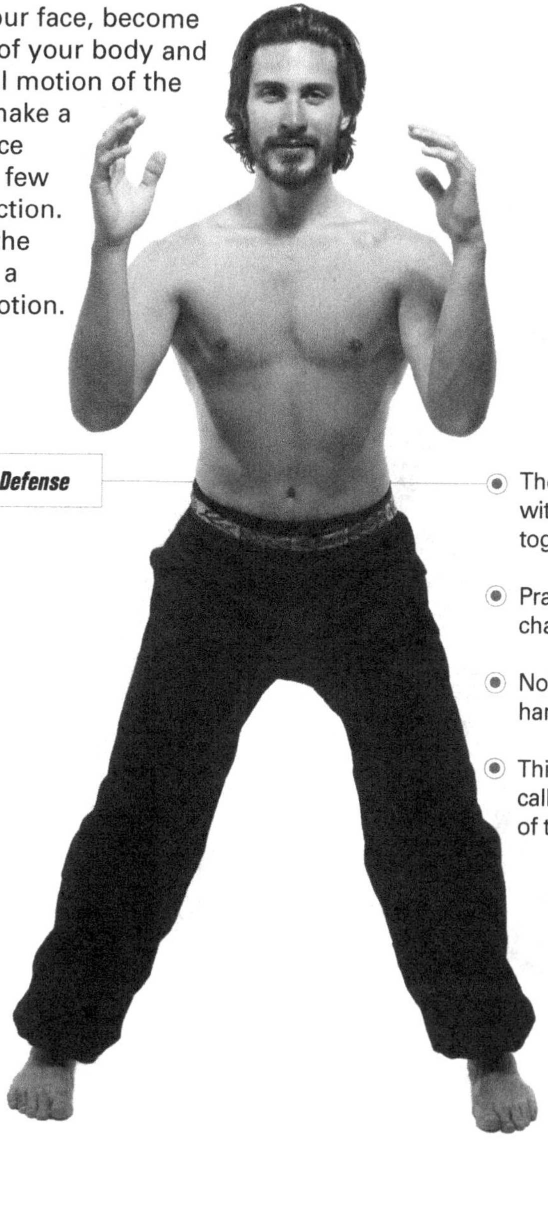

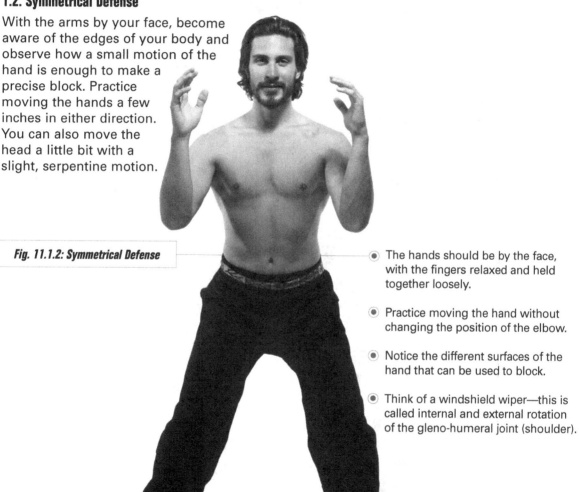

Fig. 11.1.2: Symmetrical Defense

- The hands should be by the face, with the fingers relaxed and held together loosely.
- Practice moving the hand without changing the position of the elbow.
- Notice the different surfaces of the hand that can be used to block.
- Think of a windshield wiper—this is called internal and external rotation of the gleno-humeral joint (shoulder).

1.3. Right Arm Circle Block (downward)

Maintain the symmetrical-defense position with the hands and rotate your right hand down so that it passes your face, chest, heart, and abdomen. Remember to keep the elbow steady. This defends the upper right quadrant of the body.

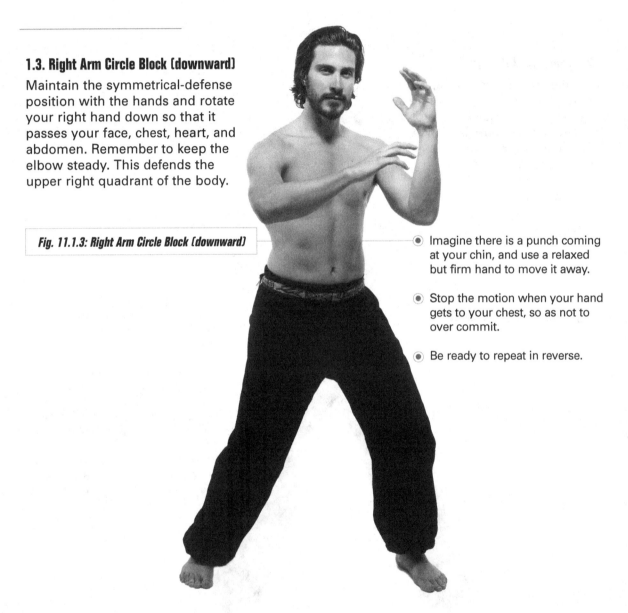

Fig. 11.1.3: Right Arm Circle Block (downward)

- Imagine there is a punch coming at your chin, and use a relaxed but firm hand to move it away.

- Stop the motion when your hand gets to your chest, so as not to over commit.

- Be ready to repeat in reverse.

1.4. Left Arm Circle Block (downward)

Keep the right arm where it is and drop the left hand to defend the upper left quadrant of the body.

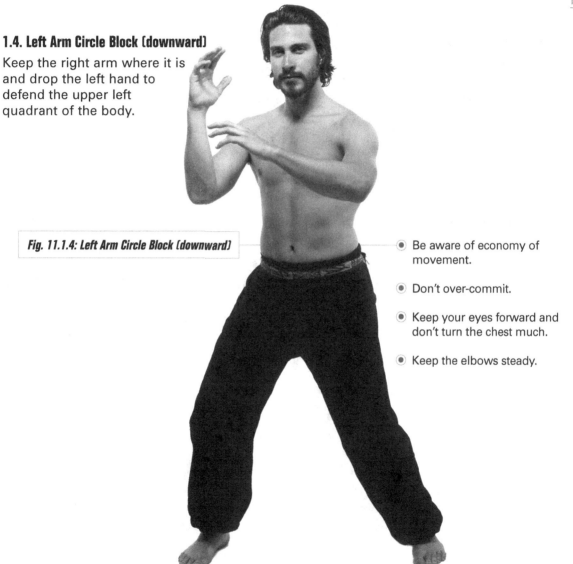

Fig. 11.1.4: Left Arm Circle Block (downward)

- Be aware of economy of movement.

- Don't over-commit.

- Keep your eyes forward and don't turn the chest much.

- Keep the elbows steady.

1.5. Right Arm Circle Block (upward)

From the defensive position, rotate your right arm to protect your face. This motion sweeps through to defend the previous areas and also the upper right quadrant of your body.

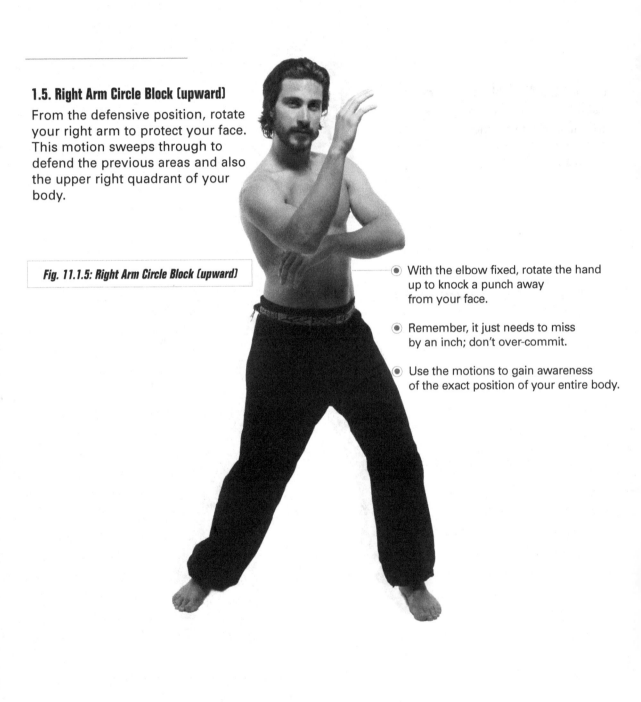

Fig. 11.1.5: Right Arm Circle Block (upward)

- With the elbow fixed, rotate the hand up to knock a punch away from your face.

- Remember, it just needs to miss by an inch; don't over-commit.

- Use the motions to gain awareness of the exact position of your entire body.

1.6. Left Arm Circle Block (upward)

Repeat the same motion with the left arm to defend the upper left quadrant.

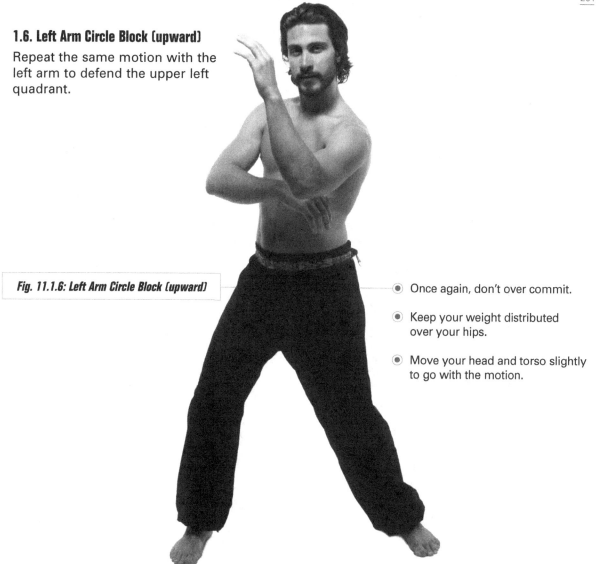

Fig. 11.1.6: Left Arm Circle Block (upward)

- Once again, don't over commit.

- Keep your weight distributed over your hips.

- Move your head and torso slightly to go with the motion.

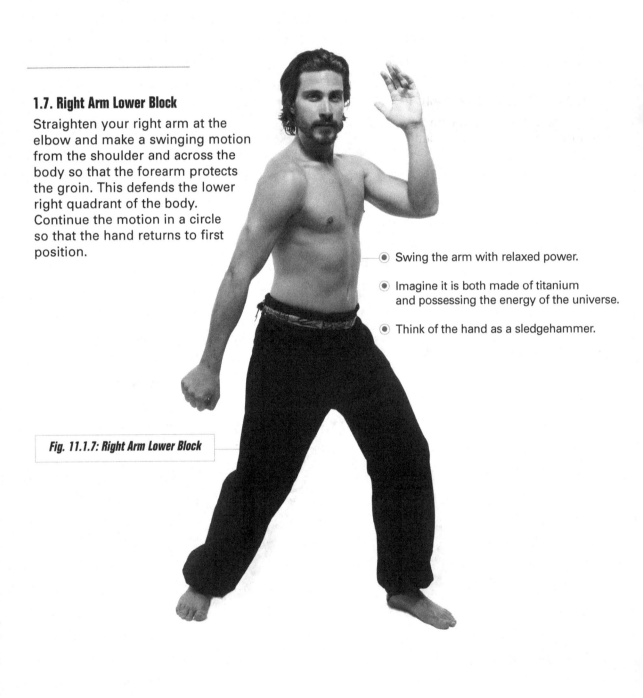

1.7. Right Arm Lower Block

Straighten your right arm at the elbow and make a swinging motion from the shoulder and across the body so that the forearm protects the groin. This defends the lower right quadrant of the body. Continue the motion in a circle so that the hand returns to first position.

- Swing the arm with relaxed power.

- Imagine it is both made of titanium and possessing the energy of the universe.

- Think of the hand as a sledgehammer.

Fig. 11.1.7: Right Arm Lower Block

1.8. Left Arm Lower Block

Swing the left arm down
to protect the left side
of the groin and
lower abdomen.

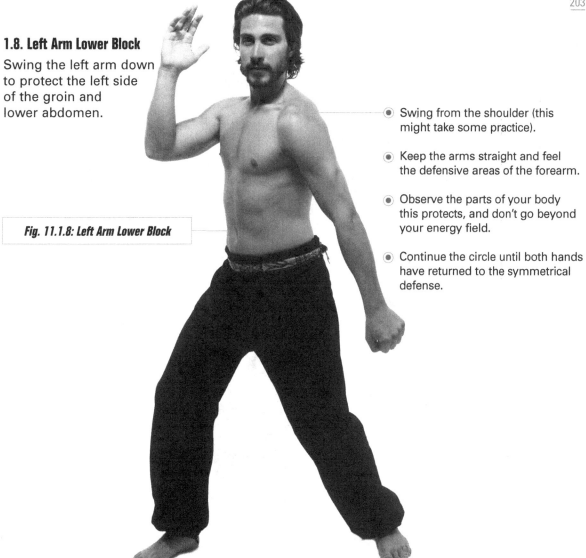

Fig. 11.1.8: Left Arm Lower Block

- Swing from the shoulder (this might take some practice).

- Keep the arms straight and feel the defensive areas of the forearm.

- Observe the parts of your body this protects, and don't go beyond your energy field.

- Continue the circle until both hands have returned to the symmetrical defense.

1.9. Right Leg Block (internal)

Remain in horse stance and shift your balance from the middle to the left leg. Turn your right leg out slightly and bend your knee, lifting the foot off the floor. Keep your knee even with the hip and rapidly bring it in so the shin sweeps across the midline. After completing the movement, place the foot back in horse stance.

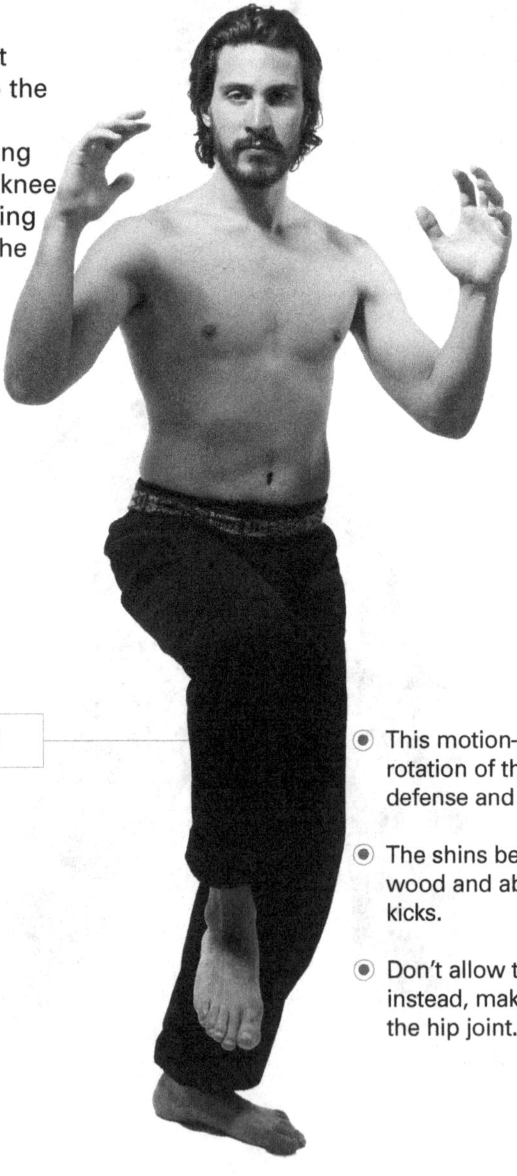

Fig. 11.1.9: Right Leg Block (internal)

- This motion—internal and external rotation of the hip—is the basis of defense and offense.

- The shins become as strong as wood and able to defend against kicks.

- Don't allow the pelvis to move much; instead, make the motion come from the hip joint.

1.10. Left Leg Block (internal)

Now shift the weight to your right leg and lift the left leg a few inches off the floor, knee bent and even with the hip. Repeat the motion. This defends the lower body against kicks.

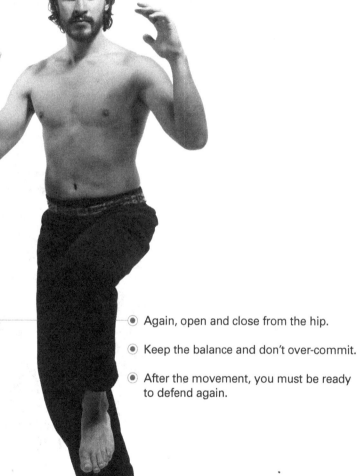

Fig. 11.1.10: Left Leg Block (internal)

- Again, open and close from the hip.

- Keep the balance and don't over-commit.

- After the movement, you must be ready to defend again.

1.11. Right Leg Block (external)

Return to the horse stance and shift the weight back onto the left leg. Bring your right leg up and close the leg inward, turning the hip slightly so that both knees are together. Then, opening from the hip, sweep the shin to the outside.

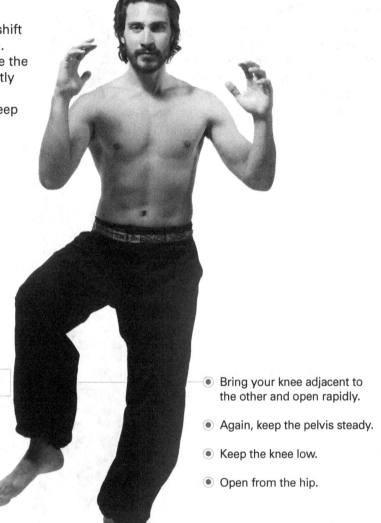

Fig. 11.1.11: Right Leg Block (external)

- Bring your knee adjacent to the other and open rapidly.

- Again, keep the pelvis steady.

- Keep the knee low.

- Open from the hip.

1.12. Left Leg Block (external)

Shift your weight to the right leg and bring your left knee adjacent to the standing leg.
Once again, open rapidly from the hip to defend the lower body with an outside sweep of the left shin.

This completes the Eight Gates. Practice this sequence in rapid succession and repeat the motions until you perform them spontaneously. Always keep your balance with slightly bent knees and your elbows as steady as possible. The rotation should come from the shoulder and not from the comparatively slow movement of the arm. Likewise, for the leg: make the motion come from a rapid opening of the hip and not from the limb. Stay rooted and balanced as you practice, but also combine your effort with poise.

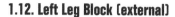

Fig. 11.1.12: Left Leg Block (external)

- Open rapidly from the knee.

- Imagine that you are blocking a kick with your shin.

- Keep your weight on the standing leg.

2. Capoeira Drills

Capoeira is a dynamic Brazilian martial art that includes musical elements, dance, and some acrobatics. Afro-Brazilian slaves developed this martial art and disguised it so they could practice without other people's knowledge. Gradually, it evolved as a cultural phenomenon, and some even think it was the forerunner to break dancing.

Capoeira probably isn't the most lethal fighting modality (that title most likely goes to Brazilian jujitsu) but capoeira is one of the most integrated practices. When played with a grin and a good community, it becomes a fun way to test your elements. Poise, flexibility, responsiveness, and timing—all combine in this multidimensional art.

What follows are some general defensive positions, which also form the basis of the *jinga*—the basic interactive motion. If you learn these as well as the Eight Gates, you will be able to learn capoeira quite rapidly. Many, if not all, of the offensive positions are derived from these defensive forms, so it is essential that you learn to coordinate the movements.

Capoeira is about poise. "Defeating" an opponent has less to do with brute strength or violence and more to do with playing a great game. It teaches you to maintain your awareness in all kinds of positions and also to lure the opponent into making a mistake. For success and safety, your moves must be accomplished with respect to the rhythm of the game. In general, you don't know *what* is going to happen, but you do have a concept of *when* something will happen. Strikes are not made in rapid succession, but on a beat; this provides structure. What you do with that beat is the inherent creativity of capoeira.

What follows are some essential defensive positions. If these catch your interest, then you can seek out a capoeira school in your area where you can participate in the circle of song, music, dance ... and a fighting spirit.

2.1. First Position

Stand in horse stance with your
arms up and drop low into your
quads for balance. Feel your body's
center and loosen up your ribcage
so you can easily move from side
to side. Because capoeira was
developed by people *who
may have been handcuffed*,
the art doesn't often employ
the arms—it relies on
the legs, acrobatics,
and flexibility.

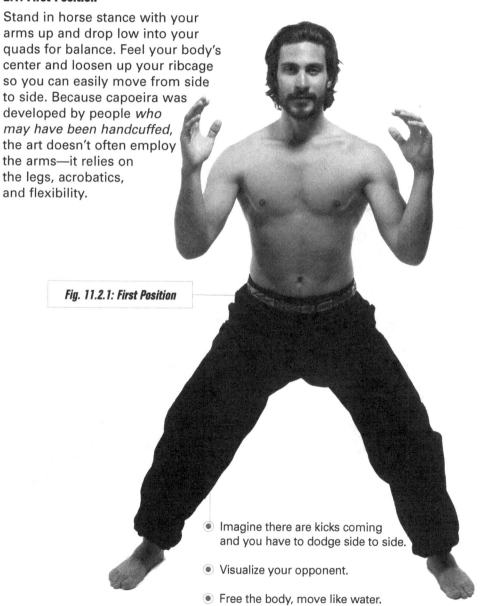

Fig. 11.2.1: First Position

- Imagine there are kicks coming
  and you have to dodge side to side.

- Visualize your opponent.

- Free the body, move like water.

2.2. Lateral Defense

Keep your hips in place and bend your body to one side, and then the other. Bring your chest down to your knee, but don't rest your hand on the floor. Keep dynamic tension in your waist, look up, and keep your elbow by your side to deflect a kick.

- Think of the side stretch from the Basic Warm-Up.

- Keep your elbows close to your body to deflect a kick.

- Keep your head up and eyes forward.

- To protect your face, keep your hand by your head.

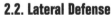

Fig. 11.2.2: Lateral Lunge

2.3. Forward Lunge

From the center position, shoot one leg back into a lunge. Keep one hand up to protect your face and lower the other hand down to touch the floor. Keep length in your back and imagine you are dropping underneath a kick.

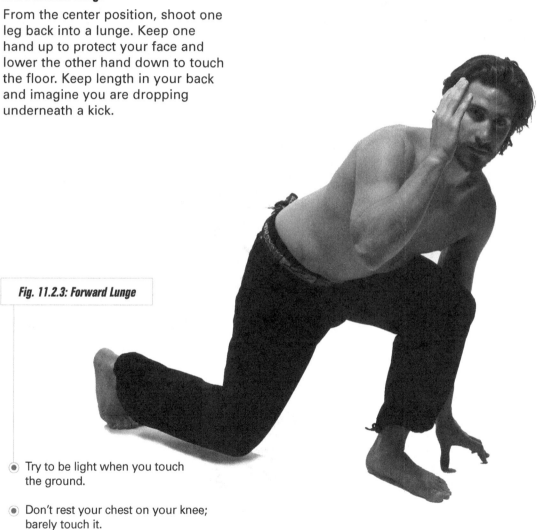

Fig. 11.2.3: Forward Lunge

- Try to be light when you touch the ground.

- Don't rest your chest on your knee; barely touch it.

- Keep your eyes up.

- Keep your weight distributed over both legs.

2.4. Posterior Lunge

Come partway up from the former position and rotate your chest back to put your weight over your back leg. You should be able to move with fluidity between this and the previous position.

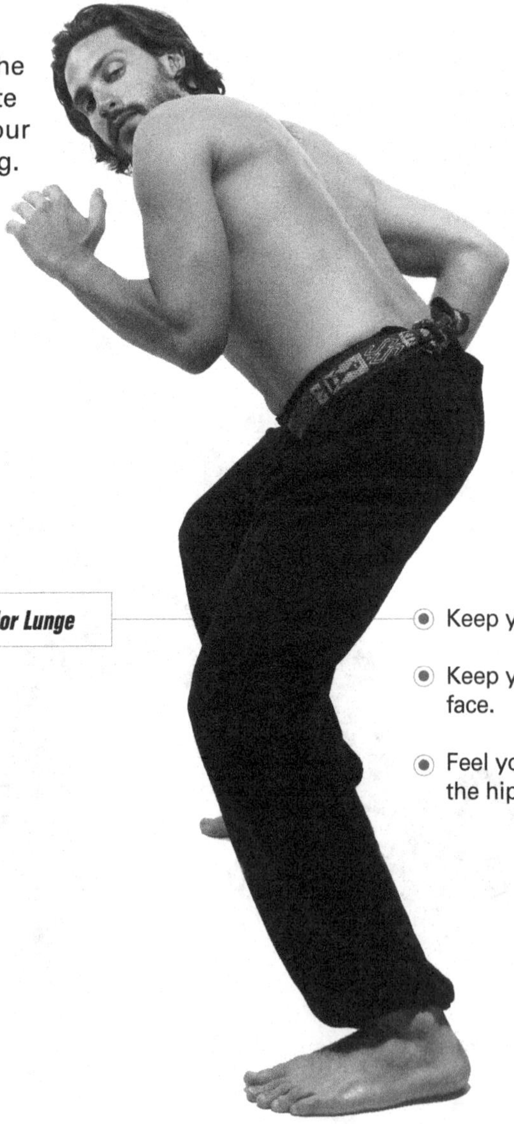

Continue to practice these exercises until you have moved into each of the four positions a minimum of five times: Start from the center and go to each side five times. Move into the forward lunge, and go from forward lunge to backward lunge five times. Next, drill in all different directions. Stay low, slow, and controlled, ever ready to defend against a strike. Practice with rhythm and relaxation. Be light on your feet and light on your hands.

Fig. 11.2.4: Posterior Lunge

- Keep your front leg slightly bent.

- Keep your arms up to protect your face.

- Feel your feet planted, but swivel from the hips.

3. CHI COIL

The chi coil is an exercise that works almost all the muscles in the arms and hands. It works the meridians of the upper body and does wonders for coordination. It can even be used as a starting point for an improvised set that includes all the elements from this chapter. This exercise begins with the hands but then connects via dynamic elasticity throughout the whole body. You will feel it in the arms, chest, back, and lats. If you do it right, you will connect to your core strength.

3.1. First Position/Pinkies Together

Return to the Basic Stance, drop your weight into the quads, and anchor your hips. Extend your hands out a bit so that the pinkies are together. Spread all your fingers evenly and let the energy move through your hands.

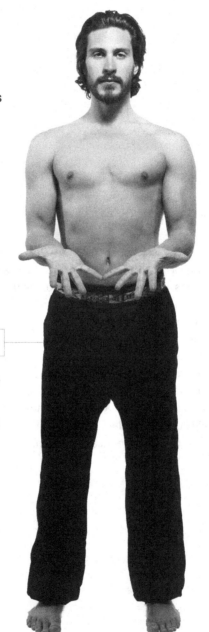

Fig. 11.3.1: First Position/Pinkies Together

- Keep equal space between each of the fingers.

- Keep the shoulders down, belly in and the chest up.

3.2. Hand Roll

Slowly rotate your hands up, pulling the energy toward you. Continue rotating until your hands are at the chest and the backs of the hands are together. Complete the rotation until the thumbs are up.

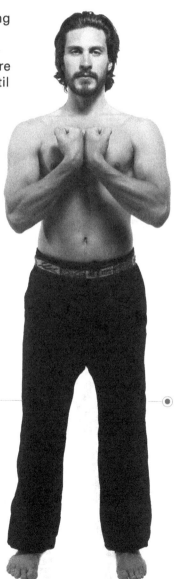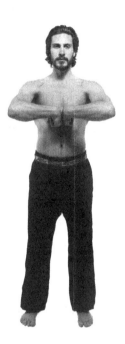

Fig. 11.3.2: Hand Roll

◉ The backs of the hands should touch and stay as close as possible to the body.

3.3. Thumbs Up/Cosmic Being

With your thumbs up, check the space between each of your fingers and energize the hands. Straighten the elbows and lift the hands to shoulder height. Slowly open your arms wide and extend through the fingers so that you end in a wide T position.

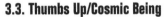

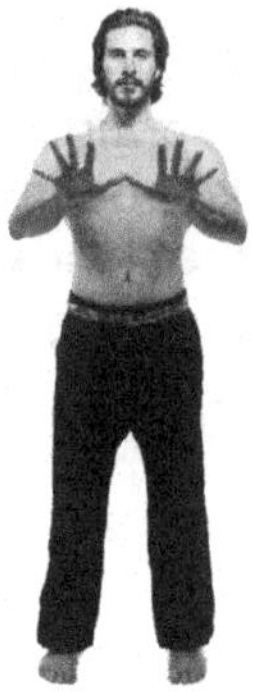

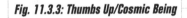

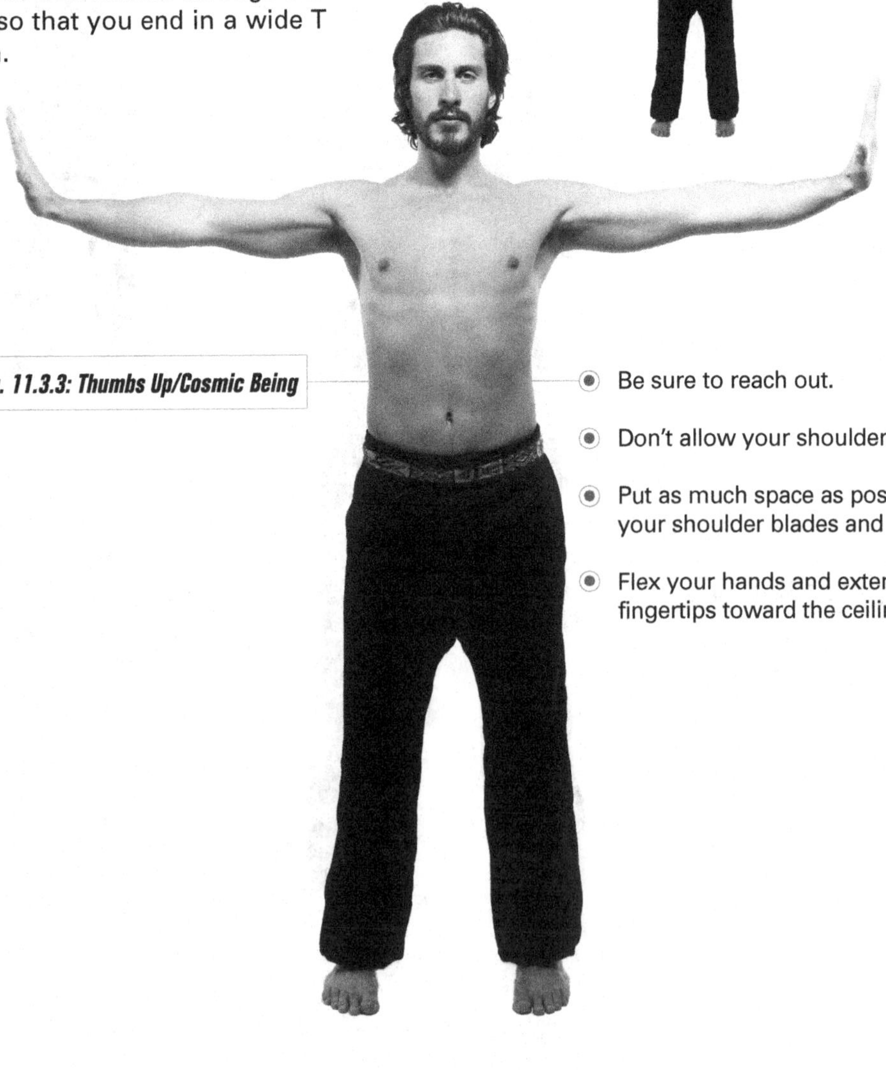

Fig. 11.3.3: Thumbs Up/Cosmic Being

- Be sure to reach out.

- Don't allow your shoulders to break back.

- Put as much space as possible between your shoulder blades and your arms.

- Flex your hands and extend your fingertips toward the ceiling.

3.4. Thumbs Together

Slowly close your arms and bring
your thumbs back together. Resume
the rotation in reverse order (downward) until the backs of your hands
come together near the chest.
Continue in this direction until you
end up with your pinkies together
again.

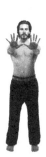

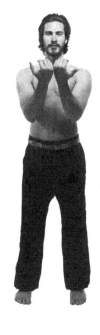

Fig. 11.3.4: Thumbs Together

- After your thumbs are together, allow
  them to lead the motion toward the earth.

- The rest of your hand follows until once
  again the backs of the hands are together.

- Complete the motion with the pinkies
  together and energize the hands.

3.5. Lat Coil

Extend through the fingers and keep energy in your arms. Check your stance, and then on inhalation, bring your hands to your sides, elbows close as if you are shaving the sides of your ribs.

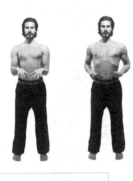

Fig. 11.3.5: Lat Coil

You have now completed one full rotation of the chi coil. This exercise cultivates internal energy. By teaching the body how to expand and release potential energy, it also helps to build the explosive energy needed for the two-inch punch. It will help prevent arthritis, tendonitis, and carpal tunnel syndrome among others. It should be practiced as an isometric exercise—with added contraction—to maximize the benefit.

- Visualize that you are absorbing chi into your body.

- You inhale not just air, but the energy of the universe.

- Gently cup your fingers to hold this energy.

4. THE DIRTY THIRTY

If, in addition to all this grace training, you want to stock up on pure strength and power; if you want definition, functionality, aesthetics, and vitality, then the Dirty Thirty is your method: Thirty push-ups, thirty straight-arm crunches or sit-ups, thirty deep squats, and thirty pull-ups. That's it, nothing but good old-fashioned boot camp. If you use your body right and make it count, there really is no need for weights; you can build plenty of muscle with resistance and your God-given kilos.

4.1. Push-Ups

There are many variations of this classic exercise. I have found two kinds to be the most effective and the least stressful on the joints.

4.1a. Pec Push-Ups

The first kind is basically a pectoral-focused push-up. The position is on the knuckles or hands with the elbows turned out slightly. Keep the whole body straight, your lower abdomen tucked, your lower back flat, your buttocks engaged, and the inner thighs squeezed together. Then lower the body down in a smooth motion.

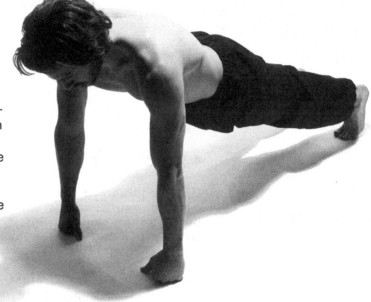

Fig. 11.4.1a: Pec Push-Ups

- Lengthen the body as much as possible.

- You can do them fast or slow, but make each one count.

- Keep energy in the feet.

- Be aware of the wrist line—keep it straight from the forearm to the knuckle.

- Don't break form.

4.1b. Triceps Push-Ups

For the second variation, maintain the same body position, but shift the weight off the knuckles. Spread the fingers and rotate the hand out slightly. Your fingers should now be pushing away from your body. Keep the elbows close by your sides and continue to squeeze the side of the body as you lower. These push-ups are primarily focused on the triceps and lats.

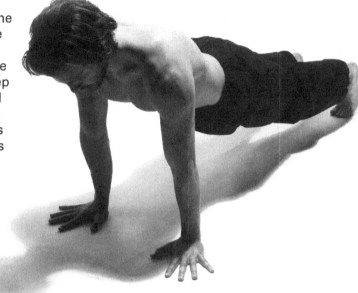

Fig. 11.4.1b: Triceps Push-Ups

● Allow yourself to lean out slightly so the shoulders are actually out in front of the arms.

● Again, keep the body straight, lengthened, and taut.

● Imagine that you are shaving the sides of your ribs with your elbows.

4.2. Deep Knee Squats

Stand with your feet shoulder-width apart. Engage the abdomen, lengthen the spine, and lift the arms in front. Then slowly and without grinding or pops, bend your knees and sit your body into a squat position. Push yourself back up and lift the heels at the top.

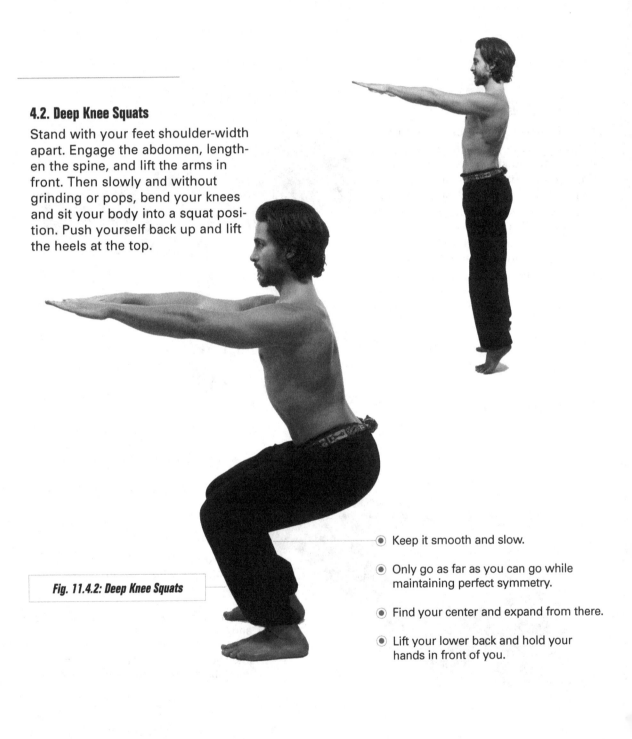

Fig. 11.4.2: Deep Knee Squats

- Keep it smooth and slow.

- Only go as far as you can go while maintaining perfect symmetry.

- Find your center and expand from there.

- Lift your lower back and hold your hands in front of you.

4.3. Over/Under Pull-Ups

Pull-Ups are one of the most effective exercises known to man—quite literally, power over gravity. Grab the bar with your left hand with your knuckles facing in (underhand grip), and grab the bar with the right hand with the knuckles out (overhand grip). Hang your body with your left knee bent. Use your abs to hold you in a position where your buttocks is slightly in front of the midline. Don't let your buttocks drop. Use your lats to connect the weight of your pelvis to the power of your shoulders. Do five (more if you can) and then switch handgrips.

> **Fig. 11.4.3: Over/Under Pull-Ups**

- Don't swing.

- Keep the buttocks and torso in front of the midline.

- Use the abs and lats to keep you stabilized.

- Squeeze the buttocks and hang the legs tight.

- Keep the face relaxed.

- Control your body.

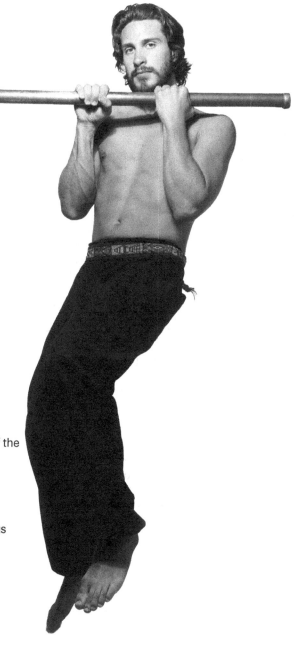

Fig. 11.5: Side Kicks

- This exercise is about balance, dynamic tension, and flexibility.

- Feel three classic directions meeting in the middle and working simultaneously: the standing leg heading downward, and the lifted leg and the torso bisecting the sky.

- Use the lateral abdominals and the lats to hold you up.

- Keep the standing leg totally straight.

5. SIDE KICKS

One last exercise that must be included is a standing leg lift. There is a famous picture of Mr. Lee holding this position, and it is much harder than it looks. To do it correctly, a dynamic chord must exist between the lateral muscles of the leg, the obliques, the core muscles, and the lats. It also demands peak flexibility from the hamstring and hip of the standing leg.

First, do a groin-stretch (see fig. 9.8) to loosen up your hips. Next, stand on one leg and lift the other one up as high as possible to the side. Put energy in the foot, flex the toes, and invert slightly so the knife-edge faces out. Use the lats and the abs to hold you up as you curl your body as much as possible to offset the leg. Push through the hip to open the quads and make one long line from the abdomen through your foot. Hold for ten seconds. Then lift and lower the leg ten times. Hold for ten more seconds. Now switch sides.

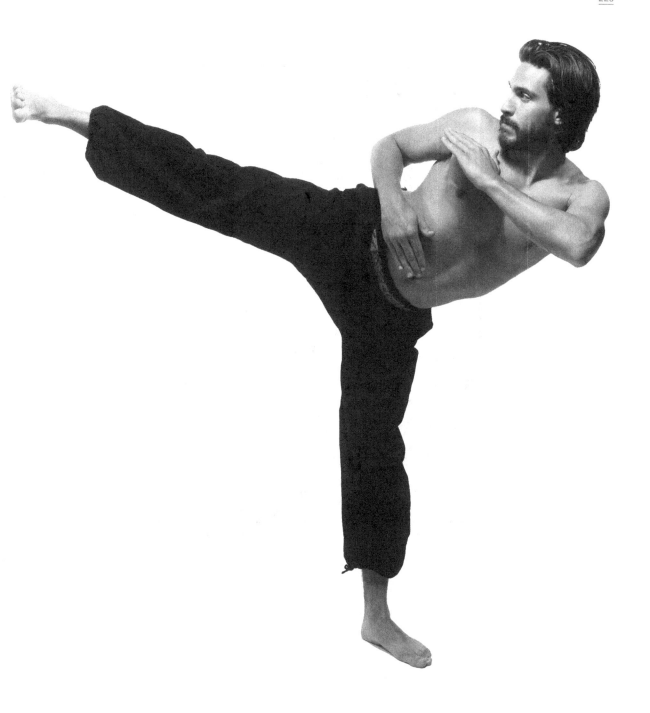

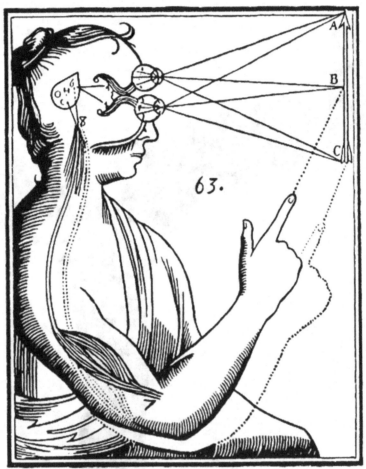

The angle of perception is the angle of reflection.

Chapter 12. *Self-Observation*

We are training to stay in the center, the circle of ease, the weightless zone. Whatever you do, let it be the training of presence. Let it be the learner that is observed—and not just the discipline. Let the discipline bring you to the master and the master in turn to universal mastery. It is between you and that, you and the universe, you and truth. You are watching the cosmic play and also the play of your individual ego as the drama unfolds before ancient and indestructible eyes—remember, you are the eyes not the movie. "In this way," promises the Bhagavad Gita, "always disciplining the self, the yogi becomes free and happily experiences the infinite bliss of union with the Brahman."*

A shepherd once approached the ancient Sufi sage, Rumi, and said, "I've been having glorious visions of God, are they true?"

Rumi replied, "Do you have a wife?"

"Yes."

"And how many children?"

"Four."

"And how many goats?"

"Forty … I'm telling you about my visions of God, and you are asking me to count my goat herd?"

Then Rumi asked, "These visions you have, do they make you a better husband and parent; do they make you kinder to every living thing?"

"Yes," the shepherd replied.

"Then I would say that they are true."

In other words, whatever works. Do what you do, and do it well. Yoga as a physical practice can become an end in itself. Yet it is an end with no end. No matter how many hours a day we practice, many of us will never achieve the most advanced postures. And the truth is, we don't need to. The average person needs a few simple things that we can do on a daily basis, and then get on with it.

Throughout this book I have presented the exercises that I believe to be the most efficient and effective for everyone. Besides improving functional strength, balance, structural integrity, the true meaning of Integrated Exercise is the practice of awareness. Becoming an artist of life. Philosophically, this is not about how many dis-ciplines you can master, nor the ability to do advanced arm-balancing, but the quest to become a master of mastery. About getting up off the mat and stepping out into the world, while retaining peace and centeredness. Who cares if you can stand on your head if you still can't parallel park your car? Awareness must be applied universally.

It's been said that we're not human beings having a spiritual experience, but rather spiritual beings having a human experience. Nevertheless, one can be an atheist and still appreciate the value of self-realization. The root goal of "awareness training" is to optimize your body to express your being. Thus it becomes possible to fully express your "soul print" or unique intelligence. Once the body has taken form, we can focus on what is most important in life. Whatever it is.

But what if we don't have any visions? Don't know what to do with our lives? What if we're doing yoga, meditation, chi kung, Reiki, Pilates and we still wake up miserable every morning? Still haven't made contact?

Something's gotta give.

In many traditions, the beginning of all cures is through fasting. When we fast, we remove ourselves from the process of thinking about food, preparing food, digesting food, eliminating food, and this allows us to tune in to the more subtle elements of thought processes and behavior. Of course, you should consult your

---

* *Brahma means universal consciousness, or God, in the Hindu tradition.*

physician first. And it may not be necessary to completely abstain from food. Refer to chapter 8 and reread the bit on cleansing or go on the Internet and find what works for you.

If you decide to cleanse, it's a good idea to take off three or four days and spend a week beforehand cleaning up your life, inside and out. Ideally, the fast is a time for rest, reflection, and healing. Though certain activities might synchronize with the restorative process of fasting: there have been times when I've channeled my extra energy into cleaning or going through papers—organizing my life, reassessing what's important, restoring order to my environment as the fast restores it to my body.

It may also help to go on a vision quest. In many traditional societies, the warriors, shamans, and healers would be sent into the woods. And they would stay there until the vision came. When we step beyond the protective shield offered by life's distractions, we step out to experience the unknown in our own heroic way. It's about contact. Real experience now, at this moment in life.

And what are we looking for? What is the holy grail? To return with new energy and clarity. Stillness. Serenity. The vision quest is a method of seeking that can lead to direct revelation—such as the answer to a question or some kind of wisdom that would aid the tribe; often it is increased self-knowledge.

It's a quest, a journey within. This means not just abstaining from food, but also from media, from the web, from the smart phone, from music, from habits of thought. What then? What to do with all that time?

TIPS FOR OPTIMIZING YOUR LIFE

1. Examine your belief system. Socrates is reported to have said that if he was the wisest man in all of Athens, it was not for what he knows, but for the fact that he knows he doesn't know. The first step to self-observation is to seek efficiency and conscious intention in all actions. It is easy to find fault in others, but far more valuable to find fault in ourselves. Not negative criticism, but pure discriminative reason: If a thought pattern disrupts this flowing and vibrant health, it must be discarded. We must enter a constant state of self-observation, because the most dangerous lies are the ones we tell ourselves. Practice admitting when you don't know something. Reconsider all assumptions. This is the path to objectivity.

2. Design your reality. Realize that choices and decisions determine the playing field of our life. Imagine you are born today. These are the cards you've been dealt. You have the capacity to attract what you focus on; therefore, place intention upon each thought. Become the director of your life rather than an extra. Sometimes I like to imagine that each day is the first day of my life. I just woke up in this body with this set of challenges. What am I going to do about it? Now. I don't want to have a bad day. Ever.

3. Educate the centers. The practice of mental efficiency spills over to movement in the world. What improvements can be made in your physical, emotional, intellectual, and spiritual life? Optimal attunement means flexibility and vibrant health on all levels. No matter how spir-

itual we are, we still must exist in a physical reality; therefore the more integrated we are, the easier it will be to play the game of life.

4. Control impressions. The flow of images, whether from TV, from porn, from radio ads, from billboards, from texting, from Wi-Fi—these are the manifestations of form, illusion, and they excite the consciousness. Enjoy if you will. But remember that just as our bodies are made up of a combination of our body type and the food we consume, our minds are made up of our inborn temperament and the images and ideas we put into it.

5. Study the essence. Whatever you call it and however it speaks to you, find a way to connect to the mystery. It can be yoga; it can be walking; it can be reading scriptures, poems, music, children, anything. But connect. Make a daily practice of contemplation in order to cultivate a feeling of reverence and gratitude, filling your mind with positive thoughts and vibrations.

6. Continue to practice. Even if we realize enlightenment, we still must participate with willful, emphatic submission and play by certain physical laws. Each day and each moment of the day lie at the root of personal reflection. The challenge is not just to attain, but also to maintain. This takes constant focus and determination.

STAY IN THE ZONE

If you want to go deeper in your practice, take a few days and get away from it all, because as long as we are busy, the water in our minds remains muddy, but when we can get time and space for stillness, the particles settle out.

The observation of consciousness allows us to distinguish between innermost being or essence and the forms or affects we've taken on in order to exist in the world. What Jung called the *persona*. It's not just about losing weight, but about letting go of what weighs us down, on all levels.

Once we are able to observe the *persona*, its unnecessary and neurotic elements start to vanish. During the fast or vision quest, one's being is pressed into a loaded experience that, without being physically dangerous, can feel psychologically *near death*, allowing us to follow the labyrinth of memories, defense mechanisms, and self-doubt to broker the soul's release from the matrix of inherited social bondages. What's left is the wisdom of the teacher within. Thus, the often-terrifying nature of the vision quest, fast, or renunciation experience allows us to safely pit ourselves against our own fears and mortality, giving an opportunity to let go of anything nonessential.

If you don't like the idea of fasting, then maybe climb a mountain, or immerse yourself in another culture's spiritual tradition as I did when I went to the Peruvian jungle and worked with an indigenous shaman and his Ayahuasca medicine brew. In reality, you don't need to go anywhere. Hafiz said, "If you want to get to know your Self, lock up in a dark closet three days without food." Once you return, you will likely have some clarity on what to do next to optimize your life.

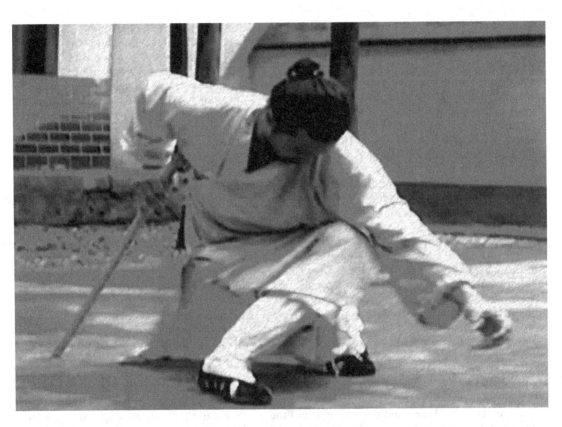

Ayahuasca is a rascal and seems to have an innate intelligence. Though invariably intense, the nice thing is that the experience always ends, and when the ceremony closes there is a sense of tranquility, humility, and excitement to embark on a new life. It always seems to answer your questions. Like an oracle. To anyone without direct, subjective experience, I understand that may sound crazy. But whatever level it works on, it will never be identified or understood by feeding it to monkeys and monitoring their brains. It cannot be known by molecules alone, only by consciousness, which is to say, by direct experience.

AFTERWORD. *Shamanic Yoga*

In December of 2006, I entered the Peruvian Amazon for a sort of vision quest: a traditional shamanic apprenticeship called a *dieta*. This would be the pinnacle of years of training and the birth of what would become this book.

After travelling up the swollen headwaters of the Amazon in a dugout canoe, I stayed in an open-air hut, ate only boiled rice and medicinal plants, and meditated on the essence of existence. Every other night, I would meet with the shaman and the other participants to sit for an *Ayahuasca* ceremony, a five-hour psychedelic meditation.

This subject may seem out of place given the context of this book (or perhaps not), but without these experiences, I doubt if I ever would have been able to develop the forms and ideas that became *Weightlessness*, or at least not until much later. In fact, while still in the jungle, I saw this project very clearly, and that vision helped me to carry it through to the end. Furthermore, as my goal for this book is to help people, it would be irresponsible of me not to share my most valuable secret. And so I must give credit where credit is due.

Ayahuasca is a powerful elixir used throughout the Amazon basin and at the root of the area's shamanic medicine tradition. It is nontoxic and only physically dangerous if mixed with certain foods.* It is fully legal in Peru as well as some other countries with indigenous populations that use it and consider it a *master plant*. In fact, shamans—or *sanadors* as they are called there—claim that it contains 90 percent of all the information in the plant kingdom. They will use it not only to gather information about the cause of a disease but also to learn the properties of other plants. The main ingredient is a jungle vine, the ayahuasca, an MAO inhibitor that can alchemize the psychoactive molecule (DMT) present in various other plants such as *chacruna* or *Psicotria viridus*. In other words, it's a psychedelic, though with a specific application and purpose. Metaphysically, ayahuasca seems to break down some of the barriers between the different levels of consciousness and will often—especially if people are harboring sickness or repressed memories—lead to vomiting, which manifests as a powerful cleansing experience.

Still, it can be a bit of a taboo in the yoga community to discuss such things. But if you've followed this book this far, you know I'm not an orthodox yogi, and I choose to conclude with this somewhat controversial subject because I believe ayahuasca (in its proper setting under the supervision of an experienced sanador) is one of the most efficient and reliable ways to shock the ego out of its slumber, especially now, when the close relationship with the guru or teacher has (often) given way to boot camp teacher trainings.

I'm not advocating psychedelics *per se*, any more than I endorse a specific style or school of yoga; and I'm certainly not supportive of taking drugs to escape, intoxicate, or get high. I am aware of the ramifications as well as the dangers, legal and otherwise, for such abuse—and that the *other-worldliness* of the experience can be terrifying. Nor is it my intention to argue the intricacies and problems of the psychedelic experience.† To state my position: I believe that research should continue and that studies such

---

*The Ayahuasca is not poisonous, but it works by inhibiting certain enzymes that normally deactivate the poisons in common foods, such as pork, dried figs, and overripe avocados. Therefore participants always follow strict dietary regulations, and consult their physicians to make sure there are no contraindications.

† Interested readers should consult *LSD: My Problem Child* by Albert Hoffman and *Cleansing the Doors of Perception* by Huston Smith. See endnotes for full citation.

as the "Good Friday Experiment"* should be repeated with the same intellectual rigor we put to other branches of science and psychology; that every attempt should be made to rebrand psychedelics as valuable substances that can be used in an appropriate context by healthy and supervised adults.

From what I have witnessed and experienced, the ayahuasca experience is like compressing five years of psychoanalysis and a forty-day fast into one night. That can be a bit extreme, which is why it is always taken with a shaman. With music and palm-fan, he or she is there to turn breakdowns into breakthroughs.

Thinking back to my first psychedelic experience, it was before I ever saw the movie *The Matrix*, but that is the best description I can offer. It was like taking the blue pill and realizing that, up until then, my life had been on some kind of autopilot. In Indian terms, this is known as *maya*, the illusion or dream of the world. Standing outside the matrix, one realizes consciousness as a holographic entity. Normally dissipated, it can become crystallized into an omnidimensional sphere—*a pilot*. For me, this was the beginning of self-awareness. Looking back on this and other clandestine consciousness research, I have never seen anything *not there* like elves, monsters, or dragons. What I have seen is a terrifyingly beautiful molecular intelligence inside my mind. I have also seen, outside, a greater awareness of patterns, color, texture. Inside: parading images from my psyche, a sense that my whole life was flowing together like a symphony, with mythological overtones; I have sensed deep compassion and empathy, moving me closer to my family, loved ones, the earth; the realization of the mask, the personal ego, and the necessity for transcendence; that my mind and body, though relatively young and healthy, were so far from human potential. Perhaps most important, I began to sense my body as an instrument and had glimpses of what can be called *cosmic consciousness*—where the personal self is dissolved into the universal mystery.

Whether, physical or metaphysical, I have invariably come out of the experience with a to-do list for my soul, body, intellect, and mind.

EMPIRICAL METAPHYSICS

The word psychedelic was coined by Aldous Huxley and Humphrey Osmond and comes from a Latin root intended to mean "psyche manifesting." This is a far more accurate term than hallucinogenic, which comes from a root meaning "to wander in the mind" and implies seeing things that aren't really there. More recently, and because the word psychedelic has bad connotations, many scholars, including Huston Smith, have begun to use the word *entheogenic*, which translates roughly to "God within generating." It is the term of choice for the responsible and ceremonial approach to psychoactive chemicals. Insofar as these substances can (in certain circumstances) help generate a *second birth* of the spiritual man out of the animal man, I would say this is an apt and accurate description.

Still, many people feel that these substances are the domain of crazed witch doctors or dazed and confused hippies. Since the sixties, main-

*Marsh Chapel Experiment: Harvard University 1962. In a double-blind study to prove whether psilocybin would act as an entheogen—substance able to create a religious experience—the control group was given niacin, which caused flushing of the face and tingling. Almost all the members of the experimental group (those given psilocybin) reported experiencing profound religious experiences, providing empirical support for the notion that psychedelic drugs can facilitate religious experiences. http://en.wikipedia.org/wiki/Marsh_Chapel_Experiment.

stream science and psychology has largely ignored what will likely prove to be one of the greatest tools of inner technology ever known. Luckily, recent studies have reopened the dialogue, and begun to acknowledge the value of such experiences. One such study, at Johns Hopkins University (2006), showed that psilocybin, the active chemical in so-called magic mushrooms (a molecule very similar to DMT, the active chemical in ayahuasca), can "under very defined conditions, with careful preparation ... safely and fairly reliably occasion what's called a primary mystical experience that may lead to positive changes in a person."[*]

The article continues to state that,

It's an early step in what we hope will be a large body of scientific work that will ultimately help people ... more than 60 percent of subjects described the effects of psilocybin in ways that met criteria for a "full mystical experience" as measured by established psychological scales. One-third said the experience was the single most spiritually significant of their lifetimes; and more than two-thirds rated it among their five most meaningful and spiritually significant ... Two months later, 79 percent of subjects reported moderately or greatly increased well-being or life satisfaction compared with those given a placebo at the same test session. A majority said their mood, attitudes, and behaviors had changed for the better. Structured interviews with family members, friends, and coworkers generally confirmed the subjects' remarks.

Do I think these "master plants" should be lawfully available to the serious student of consciousness? Yes. Do I think they violate spiritual "laws"? Not necessarily. Just like other traditions, yoga can also lapse into a type of fundamentalism, albeit a more flexible one. Besides, if all things are, as the yogis would say, Brahma, then what difference does it make? Many verses in the Vedas (ancient yogic scriptures) are actually hymns to the psychoactive substance Soma.[†] In Persia, it was the Hoama; Ayahuasca has been in use for thousands of years, and before the Judeo-Christian age, there were shamanic peoples all over the Europe and Middle East.[‡] If scientific, cultural, and empirical evidence is considered objectively, one gets the sense that entheogens may have a greater role in the formation of human culture and religions than many would like to admit. These facts are too significant to be ignored, especially by psychologists, practitioners of the healing arts, yogis, and students of consciousness.

In the words of Mary Barnard,[§]

Which was more likely to happen first? The spontaneously generated idea of an afterlife in which the disembodied soul, liberated from the restrictions of time and space, experiences eternal bliss, or the accidental discovery of hallucinogenic plants that give a sense of euphoria, dislocate the center of the consciousness, and distort time and space, making them balloon out in greatly expanded vistas? ...

---

[*] *http://www.hopkinsmedicine.org/Press_releases/2006/07_11_06.html.*

[†] *Soma is mentioned in the Rig Veda approximately 114 times and was considered a god above all others. http://en.wikipedia.org/wiki/Soma.*

[‡] *In Persia, the Soma was referred to as Hoama and was possibly an ayahuasca analogue-substance made from different plants but with similar properties to the Amazonian entheogen. It is possible to make a brew containing Syrian Rue (Peganum harmala) and a common species of Acacia.*

[§] *Mary Barnard, quoted by Huston Smith in Cleansing the Doors of Perception (Sentient Publications; 3rd ed.), April 25, 2003.*

Looking at the matter coldly, unintoxicated and unentranced, I am willing to prophecy that fifty theobotanists,* working for fifty years would make the current theories concerning the origins of much mythology and theology as out of date as pre-Copernican astronomy.

That pretty much sums it up. As William Blake says, "If the doors of perception were cleansed, then mankind would see the Universe as it is, infinite."

Or in Huxley's† words:

The mescaline experience is without any question the most extraordinary and significant experience available to human beings this side of the Beatific Vision. To be shaken out to the ruts of ordinary perception, to be shown for a few timeless hours the outer and inner worlds, not as they appear to an animal obsessed with survival or to a human being obsessed with words and notions, but as they are apprehended, directly and unconditionally by Mind at Large—this is an experience of inestimable value to anyone.

Yoga, if defined as the "intentional stopping of the unintentional chatter of the mind," is a natural fit, a complement for the integration and assimilation of such visions. Even Pattanjali, in his sutras, acknowledges that "psychic powers" can be accessed either because of practice, past lives, or the ingesting of certain plants. And it can certainly be argued that the explosion of yoga and Eastern thought was a direct consequence of the 1960s, when LSD was commonplace especially in creative, intellectual, and artistic communities. Unfortunately, the "court jester" of the movement, Timothy Leary, was fond of saying, "Turn on, tune in, drop out"—this formula is missing the fourth part: return.

As I write this, it has been more than five years since I have ingested any such substances. As Huston Smith says, "When you get the message, hang up the phone." It is true that people absolutely can get *there* without any assistance whatsoever, there is no substitute for discipline and practice, and the doors are open to all, but I don't consider the entheogenic sacrament as cheating any more than it is cheating to use a telescope to look at the stars. Regardless, stargazing, without star-mapping, will not make one an expert in astronomy; and one must make every effort to do the work—meditation, contemplation, intellectual, spiritual, physical and emotional development—that is necessary to transform ideals into reality, states into stages.

Although the psychedelic experience is often revealing, heart wrenching, and severe as a Zen master, nothing terrible happened to me, and ultimately when I came down, I experienced a partial ego-death. The part of me that had suffered, feared, and felt anxiety, was the only thing that could suffer, fear, and feel anxiety: my limited, partial, egoic self. Maya, illusion.

Now back to the Amazon ...

THE COSMIC SERPENT

Alone in the jungle, with just a mosquito net, a hammock, and a hard, thin mattress, you get to know yourself; you learn about work and love. On the first day, I noticed a bird's nest that was next to the hut and waist high in a tree. Later on, a small brown bird returned to it and laid two eggs there. The nest was less than a body's

---

* *Theobotanist: one who ingests psychoactive plants in a ceremonial context.*
† *Aldous Huxley as quoted by Huston Smith in* Cleansing the Doors of Perception *(Sentient Publications; 3rd ed.), April 25, 2003.*

length from my bed, and I hoped that, before I left, I would see the hatchlings. It could have been any bird in any forest in the world, but this one was special to me—the eggs became a symbol of new life and of the triumph of life over death.

Before each ceremony, I had set a question or intention, in yogic terms, a sankalpa. Think of ayahuasca like inviting a master chef to your house—under the condition that you will buy the ingredients. Even a master chef can only do so much with bread and almond butter. So it is up to you to stock the fridge. This is what I mean by "setting an intention." You can do the same for your day, every day.

The first ceremony had revealed to me that my body was fundamentally healthy and that I was in a good relationship with my parents. The second revealed that the woman (who is now my life partner) would be what she has become. In fact, those two eggs were omens of the two beautiful children that we now have. The third ceremony revealed to me my work as a writer and practitioner of the healing arts. Specifically, the visualization of this book, and a forthcoming novel called *The Medicine*.* That was it. Work. Love. Health. What else? After the third ceremony, I practiced the four forms—warm-up, eight brocades, sun salute, and swimming dragon—and felt the healthiest I have ever felt in my life.

As the jungle days passed from morning to twilight and then to the pitch-black night, these exercises kept me at ease, kept my spine lengthened and my head clear.

As you are away from intoxicants, stimulants, salt, perfume, even processed soap, all the senses come alive. There, in those jungle nights,

after meditating and practicing, I could hear once again the sound of the universe and experience periods of unbroken awareness. My ears followed the animals and crickets, the wind and the leaves and the rain, until I was listening to existence itself. And it seemed to be an enchanted cosmic womb. Again, the beautiful sound of the *Aum*. I rested in transcendence, feeling a tremendous sense of peace, but also couldn't wait to get out, to return to my love, and begin my work, sharing these exercises with the world.

In between ceremonies, I also spent many hours sitting with and listening to the bird, and at some point each day, I would explore. On the morning of the fourth ceremony, I ventured deep into the forest, and I felt I went back in time, to a primal mind. All around me I could hear birds, insects, howler monkeys, and I could feel my body at last moving like an ancient—like an animal, supple, fluid, soft, strong. I can honestly say that it was the most perfect feeling I've ever had. When I returned to my hut, the shaman came and told me it was time for a ceremony. I told him that I felt I had learned what was necessary and didn't want to participate. He looked me in the eyes and said that it would break the spirit of the group—there was still more to see. So I agreed. This time, I set my intention to learn more about literature, which ultimately is about humanity and conflict.

I dressed and made my way to the thatched temple to sit and drink the medicinal tea, but as time passed and I looked around, I was overwhelmed by the sickness in the other participants. I recognized it from my clients. From posture. From breath and facial expressions. Now the people were really getting into it. The depth

---

* To read a sample chapter, go to www.rayrizz.com/literature.html.

of their sickness rising up, contorting their faces and spines. *Just let go*, I thought. *Let it all go*. Sit straight, breathe, and pay attention. That was it.

But what of my own sickness? I'd purged ten times previously, so I prepared with a proper diet, and for the first time, everything was all right in my tummy. I could empathize with the others, but many of them seemed to be holding onto a deep sense of fear that had become character armor, disease, and distortion—what Wilhelm Reich called the "plague of man." And they were guarding it like Gollum in *Tolkien's Lord of the Rings*. In the *Murder of the Christ*,* Reich writes,

The myth of Jesus Christ presents the qualities of God, in other words of the unborn naturally given life energy, in a nearly perfect manner. What it does not know, or recognize, is that evil, or the devil, is a perverted god grown out of the suppression of the god-like. This lack of knowledge is one of the cornerstones of the human tragedy.

This type of sickness is the hardest to cure. But the ayahuasca seems to pull it out of us like a drawing salve. Fear. Suffering. Resentment. But only if you have the courage to sit up and, as the shaman would say, *face the ayahuasca*. There in the octagonal temple, with the jungle sounds all around, participants would struggle to sit up, to quiet the mind. To let go. Yet as the ceremony progressed, some were descending into the underworld.

Then like that, the music changed. The shaman came over, tapping one woman with the palm fan. She was acting out, her soul completely transparent; though well into her fifties she was suddenly reliving a childhood neurosis; it

hadn't been *caused* by the ayahuasca; it was just being manifested and revealed. As she descended into the episode, she began to weep uncontrollably, reliving her resentment of her parents; then, facing it, she finally had the courage to purge. When it was through, something was visibly lifted. For my part, I had found a center and was trying to focus on inner experiences, but kept getting pulled away by the others. The shaman noticed this and came to my side, "You can return to your tombo if you wish," he said, tapping me on the shoulder.

I folded my blanket and pawed off barefoot into the jungle, leaving the temple and the ceremony in the twilight. I didn't know it at the time, but my ego had come back. It was saying, "What a good boy you are; look how straight you sit, how good you feel. Look how you made it out." Dangerous.

I was exhausted when I returned to my hut, but as I passed the tree, the bird flew off in a panic. Then, in the distance, I could hear the muted machine roar and whine of a chainsaw. It seemed to cut through my heart, sending a wave of sickness and compassion. I could also hear the moans and toil of the other participants. After days of living in absolute bliss, I felt my mind slipping back into the darkness that is our collective insanity. Almost simultaneously, I began to feel a weight, a depression. Now it wasn't my own sickness, but the sickness of the human condition.

A trickster voice whispered in my ear, "You can't escape the pain of existence. All life is suffering." When I closed my eyes, I saw snakes, an endless Gordian knot of them. And for the first time I asked, So what if I made it out? What about the rest? Truth is, I had come to the jungle

*Wilhelm Reich, The Murder of the Christ (Farrar, Straus and Giroux), New York, 1963.

for answers and was on a sabbatical from teaching, thinking I would just focus on fiction and music and distance myself from the healing arts. But now my conscience was saying something else. And having turned my back on human suffering, I was now witnessing it in cosmic proportions. I can hardly begin to explain the feeling of compassion and disappointment that punched a hole in my chest. This is when the vision came.

I thought about the traumatized earth, the Holocaust, cancer, famine, and human frailty. All life seemed to be a monster, as evidenced by a passage from the Bhagavad Gita: "And seeing Your mouths, terrible with their many rows of teeth, which resemble the destructive flames of time, I lose my sense of direction and obtain no tranquility. O God of gods, Pervader of the Cosmos, be merciful!"

Now my own courage was fading. Worn down by weeks of fasting and solitude, it was almost too much to bear … In a second, my mind flipped and the jungle went from paradise to hell. I could hear all around me the sounds of the struggle, the brutal earth, life living on life, and the sounds of my comrades, clinging to their suffering. For the first time, I thought I understood the human predicament—it was the same throughout time—it was the battle for survival, for Life to remain vital in the face of not just death and disease but also emotional trauma, stress, the cold fear of mortality that grips our spines and locks our minds.

The frantic spinning of the world like a million shamans with fans. Presently, there was a battle inside my spine between depression and elevation, between gravity and weightlessness. What the poets used to call mysterium tremendum et fascinans—the fearful and fascinating mystery.

And just when I thought I would succumb to my emotions and be devoured by the reality of death and disease, and that my spine would once again collapse like another fallen angel, I stood up and began to move, my body intuitively taking the shape of the eight brocades form. I felt the space between each of my vertebra increase, the cerebral spinal fluid flow, and at last, my energy shook off the sadness.

After finishing the form I sat down to meditate. A beautiful light like a web of diamonds exploded in my third eye, and I felt a glowing in my solar plexus. Love. *Amor Radiante*. After years of study and practice in Eastern traditions, this was the first time that I could also appreciate the beauty of the Christ image, the idea that "God" would send his only son to redeem human suffering. It wasn't about becoming a Christian, nor about a Christ complex, nor even about believing in god, but just about resonating with the notion, with the myth, that love and service were ways that we could transcend this fallen world of death and disease. Compassion. What was the sense of union or cosmic consciousness if I was still living only for myself?

Despite it all, life has meaning: To connect with the Master within. To give birth to a miniature Sun/Son or spark of life in our spiritual heart. And then to play with all you've got. With that realization, I felt once again able to participate in the suffering of the world, yet to align with the Tao, the great ultimate, and make a pledge to return to do everything that I could to help. However big, however small. And so I offer to you this book. In fact, having seen the universe stripped to its atrocious essence, that was the only thing worth living for, that and the children I would have, the romantic and infinite love that we all can find.

POST SCRIPT

Let's imagine that the real self is what looks out with our eyes. This seer can be identified as the eternal spark, visualized and realized as a bodiless witness. If, as the old quote says, "God is an intelligible sphere whose circumference is nowhere and center is everywhere," then the Self is the unique center, the perceiving I. This visualization is consistent with what Vedic philosophy would call the Atman, the indwelling spark of the great Brahman.

What if we are gods, and we tire of infinity and decide to incarnate in time, under condition of amnesia and embedded in our brainstems? The illusion of duality provides the perfect setting for human experience—a welcome relief from eternity. This whole game, all the suffering, trials, beauty, and loss is our fall; our descent into matter and into the sheath of a body to experience being alive.

To sense, touch, feel, love, eat, dance …

To allow the universe to become aware of itself … And if you accept immortality within this matrix, if you recover the ancient indestructible soul, then you beat the game, recover your memory, and the doors of perception swing wide open to reveal the ineffable mystery, the beatific vision of the whole shebang.

Still, we have this physical form. More than mantras and metaphysics, or even entheogens, it was the exercises that saved me in the jungle—that and the direct knowledge of transcendence. It was the ability to lift my spine, to sit straight, and breathe that triumphed over the recognition of the cosmic tragedy, allowing me to see through to the beyond. This same battle takes place every day of our lives.

Above all else, remain lifted.

DEEPENING YOUR PRACTICE

To learn more about the exercises and ideas presented in Weightlessness; *for workshops and booking information, or to order the companion DvD, please visit www.rayrizz.com*

RAY RIZZO *was born in New York in 1980. At the age of eight years old he fell off a cliff and injured his skull. From that point onward he suffered from headaches, and occasional visionary states. But at the age of seventeen he began to study yoga and to prac-tice austerities such as fasting, meditation, and to record his visions as poems. After several months of practice, the chronic symptoms were gone and he had discovered the ability to assist others in their healing process. To better serve this cause, he became licensed in massage ther-apy and piloted a degree program*

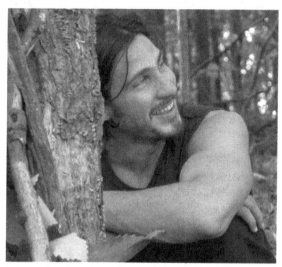

at the State University of New York in consciousness studies and holistic health sciences, working closely with Stephen Larsen to study the works of Joseph Campbell (psychology and shamanism) and performing spoken-word with the likes of Ainsley Burroughs and Simone Felice. Later, he would venture deep into the Amazon to work with traditional healers, to India, the Middle-East, China and beyond. He now practices a synthesis of healing arts through yoga, Chi kung, osteo-massage, and acupressure (LMT, CAMT). Besides being certified in the above disciplines, he was recently recognized by the Yoga Alliance as an ERYT-200 and is a graduate of Dharma Mittra's advanced 500-hour teacher training. He continually seeks to deepen his connection to the universe, and to advise others on how to connect to the power of their own wisdom through work-shops and teacher training seminars, as well as writing fiction, spoken word and hip hop. He lives in Istanbul and New York.

ILLUSTRATIONS

With the exception of those listed below, all images are photos of the author or the author's own calligraphy based on diagrams from the Taoist canon, representing longevity and liberation.

Introduction
1. Dendrite Fractal at the beginning of each chapter, by Alexis Mnnerot-Dumaine (www.wikipedia commons.webarchive/dendritejulia.png).
2. Fibonacci Sequence. Wikipedia Commons (http://upload.wikimedia.org/wikipedia/commons/thumb/9/93/Fibonacci_spiral_34.svg/1000px.jpg).
3. Persian Digestive System by Mansur Ibn Muhammad Ahmad, availlable at (www.wikipediacommons.webarchive/17th century Persian digestive system)

Chapter 1.
3. Chakra Diagram. Wikipedia Commons (http://commons.wikimedia.org/wiki/File:Chakrasss.jpg).
4. Caduceus (http://en.wikipedia.org/wiki/File:Caduceus.svg).
5. Yin Yang (http://en.wikipedia.org/wiki/File:Yin_and_Yang.svg).
6. Acupuncture Chart (http://upload.wikimedia.org/wikipedia/commons/c/cd/Acupuncture_chart_300px.jpg).

Chapter 12.
6. Pineal Gland. Rene Descartes (http://en.wikipedia.org/wiki/File:Descartes_mind_and_body.gif).

REFERENCES

Below are some of my favorite books that either directly or indirectly influenced and inspired the creation of *Weightlessness*.

1. The Bhagavad Gita: The Song of God, by Swami Prabhavananda, Christopher Isherwood and Aldous Huxley (Signet Classics), New York, 1972.
2. The Gift, Poems by Hafiz (Penguin Compass), New York 1999.
3. The Illuminated Rumi, by Coleman Barks (Broadway Books), New York, 1997.
4. The Perennial Philosophy, by Aldous Huxley (Perenial Library), New York, 1990.
5. The Power of Myth, by Joseph Campbell (Anchor), New York, 1991.
6. The Sufis, by Idries Shah (Anchor), New York, 1971.
7. The Master Game, by Robert DeRopp (Gateway Books), Nevada 1968.
8. The Murder of the Christ, by Wilhelm Reich (Farrar, Straus and Giroux), New York, 1963.
9. The Tao of Jeet Kun Do, by Bruce Lee (Ohara Publications), California, 1974.